# FRONTIER
# MEDICINE
## AT
# FORT DAVIS
## AND OTHER ARMY POSTS

# FRONTIER MEDICINE

## AT

# FORT DAVIS

### AND OTHER ARMY POSTS

. . . . . . . . . . . . . . . . . . . . . . . . . . . . . . . . . . . . . . . . . . . . . . . . . . . . . . . . . .

## TRUE STORIES OF
## UNGLAMOROUS MALADIES

### DONNA GERSTLE SMITH

THE
History
PRESS

Published by The History Press
Charleston, SC
www.historypress.com

Copyright © 2022 by Donna Gerstle Smith
All rights reserved

*Front cover (detail)*: Green U.S. Army Medical Department insignia worn on uniform sleeves of hospital stewards. *Photo by Max Kandler.*

*Opposite*: Prucha, *A Guide to the Military Posts of the United States, 1789–1895.*

First published 2022

Manufactured in the United States

ISBN 9781467152464

Library of Congress Control Number: 2022939477

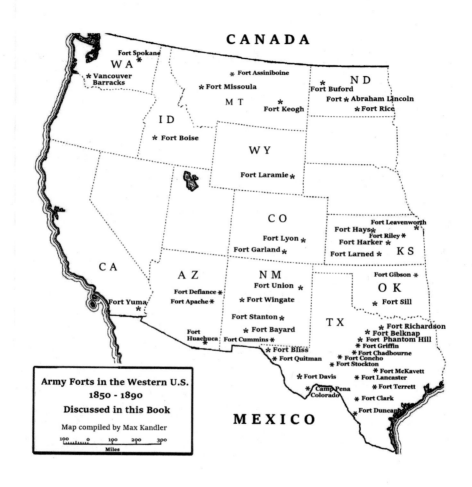

CANADA

Fort Spokane *
WA *
* Vancouver
Barracks

* Fort Assiniboine

* Fort Missoula

MT

* Fort Buford

ND

Fort * Abraham Lincoln

* Fort Keogh

* Fort Rice

ID

* Fort Boise

WY

Fort Laramie *

CO

Fort Leavenworth

Fort Hays *

* Fort Riley *

Fort Lyon *

Fort Harker *

Fort Garland *

Fort Larned *

KS

CA

AZ

NM

Fort Gibson *

Fort Defiance *

Fort Union *

OK

Fort Apache *

* Fort Wingate

* Fort Sill

Fort Yuma *

Fort Stanton *

* Fort Bayard

TX

* Fort Richardson

Fort
Huachuca *

Fort Cummins *

* Fort Belknap
* Fort Phantom Hill

* Fort Bliss

* Fort Griffin

* Fort Quitman

* Fort Chadbourne
* Fort Concho
* Fort Stockton

* Fort Davis

* Fort McKavett
* Fort Lancaster

* Camp Pena
Colorado

* Fort Terrett

* Fort Clark

MEXICO

* Fort Duncan

Army Forts in the Western U.S.
1850 - 1890
Discussed in this Book
Map compiled by Max Kandler
100    0    100    200    300
Miles

*Further Reading*

Prucha, *A Guide to the Military Posts of the United States, 1789–1895.*

# CONTENTS

# ACKNOWLEDGEMENTS

Without the kind support of family, friends, colleagues and helpful staff at various institutions, this book could never have become a reality—the author extends sincere gratitude to all. Appreciation also goes out to the people long dead whose lives are chronicled in this book—they *lived* the stories.

# INTRODUCTION

**A** walk through time—that's what this is. These true stories are just snippets of history. Many details have been lost in time. Working as a ranger at Fort Davis National Historic Site, I found that park visitors loved to hear real accounts about people who once lived—including what they suffered and sometimes died from.

This book is a compilation of honest-to-goodness, genuine stories gleaned from the real stuff of history: army records, medical reports, journals, old letters and memoirs.

Enjoy the journey traveling back to America's western frontier in the 1800s! Read on and find out:

➤ Who was the Strangling Angel of Death? (Chapter 4)

➤ How did women prevent pregnancy? (Chapters 8 and 9)

➤ What was a *magic lantern*? (Chapter 10)

➤ What did people do without toilet paper? (Chapter 11)

➤ What was a popular outdoor sport? (Chapter 12)

➤ Why was one soldier buried headless? (Chapter 15)

➤ What does *4-F* mean? (Chapter 17)

➤ Who is the Devil among the Tailors? (Chapter 23)

➤ What was in every surgeon's closet? (Chapter 28)

➤ Did parents give their kids cocaine or opium? (Chapters 32 and 33)

➤ What was *softening of the brain*? (Chapter 43)

➤ Why did the army burn down its hospitals? (Chapter 44)

# CHAPTER 1

# LET THE DEAD PEOPLE TALK

Life on the frontier was far from easy. People died, and their stories were lost… but some have descendants around to tell their stories.

As long as I live, I will never forget the day in 2007 when a man in his late eighties ambled slowly into the park visitor center. With a twinkle in his eye, he told me—the park ranger on duty—that his father was born at Fort Davis while it was still an active army post. "Say what, sir? The army closed the Fort Davis garrison in 1891. You must be mistaken."

Amazingly, he had proof to give the park: photos, military documents and an ornate marriage certificate showing that the Fort Davis post chaplain married his grandparents on March 15, 1886. They were hospital steward Richard Dart and Rachel Hetherington. He was twenty-nine, and she was twenty-one. She worked as a hospital matron/laundress.

Their son Richard Clendenin Dart—the old man's father—was born nine months later, in January 1887. By checking the post surgeon's records in the park library, I was able to confirm the birth. Army surgeon Paul Clendenin delivered the baby.

So, I gave the elderly man a tour of the hospital. He was overjoyed. He walked around quietly inside the musty building, which creaked and moaned with the wind outside. It was as if he were trying to inhale memories, to soak up a bit of history from bygone days.

For a while, he seemed to be in another world, almost like in a sci-fi movie today where someone is transported to a different time. Then he walked away in silence—satisfied to finally visit the place where his father was born

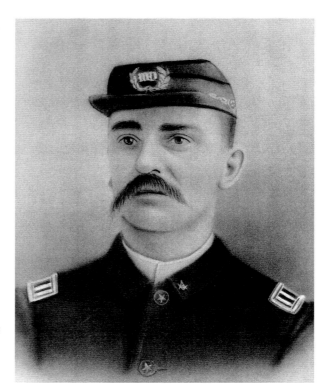

*Right*: Richard Dart/ Dare was hospital steward at Fort Davis 1885–87. He later graduated from medical school and became an army surgeon. *Fort Davis National Historic Site (hereafter NHS)*.

*Below*: Fort Davis post hospital. Two-story building (right) is hospital steward's quarters, finished early 1887. Before then, the hospital steward lived in a room at the hospital. *Lauderdale, Yale University, Beinecke Library*.

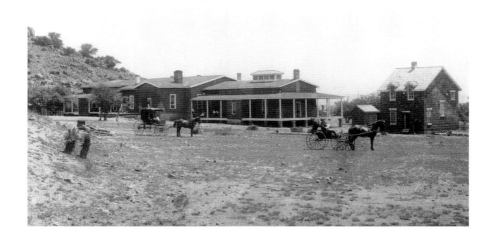

in 1887. As the park was currently restoring and partially furnishing the historic post hospital, perhaps it seemed almost alive to him.

Coming out of his daydream, he explained that his grandfather—a Canadian by birth and a druggist by training—was twenty-six when he enlisted in the U.S. Army in Boston in 1882. Since people had trouble saying his surname with the proper French pronunciation, he changed the spelling for a while from "Dart" to "Dare."

After working at several western posts, including Fort Davis, the hospital steward attended medical school, graduating in 1888 from the St. Louis College of Physicians and Surgeons. Sadly, however, he died in 1894, in his late thirties—leaving behind his wife and two small children.

It was a privilege in 2007 to meet the spunky senior citizen named Mr. Richard "Dick" Dart. Just being with him was awe-inspiring. He had traveled with a nephew many miles to visit Fort Davis, where his father was born 120 years earlier.

Without knowing it, the gentleman had allowed me to touch history in a palpable way. Truly unforgettable!

## Further Reading

Richard "Dick" Dart, author interview, 2007; communication with his nephew Mike Kennedy, Colorado, 2007.

## CHAPTER 2

# STEP BACK IN TIME

**W**e are time travelers—stepping back to open doors long closed, to unravel mysteries, to understand and honor the lives of those who came before us. Life expectancy in America in 1900 was only forty-seven years; for Black people, it was only thirty-three years.

Medical stories like those in this book pique our curiosity and give us insight into a time not so long ago. It's the best way to bring history to life: let the old souls tell how it happened.

For the dead to tell their stories, we sometimes use primary resources, such as old letters and timeworn army medical records. Within the hallowed walls of the National Archives in Washington, D.C. are fragile nineteenth-century medical registers, handwritten exams of applicants aspiring to be U.S. Army doctors 170 years ago and crumbling documents yellowing with time.

In files of people long dead are letters written with quill pens dipped in ink; some are in bundles fastened with silk ribbons. Untying dainty ribbons tied over a century ago is like peering into the spirits of the dead. Many stories could not be told without such time-worn paper documents.

Some of the stories are fascinating just because of the names—like the thirty-year-old soldier treated at the Fort Davis post hospital for a headache in 1880. His name was Eggnog Cloudy, or maybe Eggnog Chardy—old handwriting can be difficult to decipher. He was sent back to the barracks, where he remained under treatment for four days. It is not recorded what the army doctor gave Private Eggnog for his headache. Popular remedies at the time included arsenic, ammonia, cyanide of potassium, *eau sedatif,*

# FORCEPS FOR THE EXTRACTION OF ARROW-HEADS.

## By J. H. BILL, M.D.,

### SURGEON U. S. ARMY.

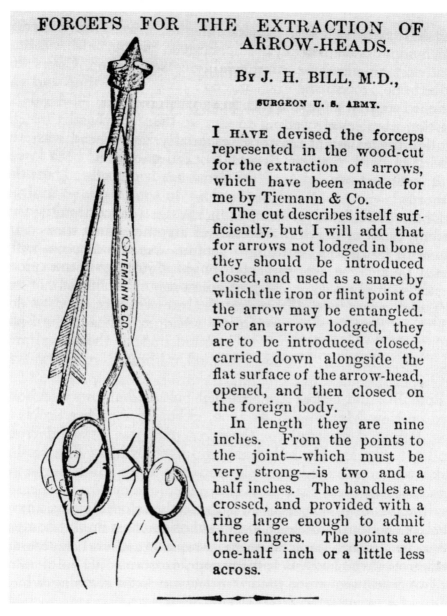

I HAVE devised the forceps represented in the wood-cut for the extraction of arrows, which have been made for me by Tiemann & Co.

The cut describes itself sufficiently, but I will add that for arrows not lodged in bone they should be introduced closed, and used as a snare by which the iron or flint point of the arrow may be entangled. For an arrow lodged, they are to be introduced closed, carried down alongside the flat surface of the arrow-head, opened, and then closed on the foreign body.

In length they are nine inches. From the points to the joint—which must be very strong—is two and a half inches. The handles are crossed, and provided with a ring large enough to admit three fingers. The points are one-half inch or a little less across.

Dr. J.H. Bill's tong-like arrowhead-removing instrument. He stressed the importance of removing arrowhead and shaft as one piece. *From Joseph Howland Bill*, The Medical Record: A Weekly Journal of Medicine & Surgery, *April 8, 1876.*

nitrate of amyl, a fungus called ergot that grows on grasses like rye, as well as galvanism—applying an electric current to tissues. (Aspirin did not come on the market until the late 1890s.)

Another true story tells of an army surgeon, Ebenezer Swift, MD, who used a rather odd tool for an emergency medical procedure. In the 1850s, a soldier was bathing in the creek near Fort Chadbourne, Texas, when he was shot in the back with an arrow by a Native American. The terrified man went running naked to the garrison with the arrow sticking out of his shoulder blade. Luckily, the arrow shaft had no arrowhead, but Dr. Swift found the arrow so firmly stuck in the soldier's bone that his case of medical instruments contained nothing adequate for the job. So, he used blacksmith's tongs—no doubt hastily borrowed from the army's blacksmith shop. Dr. Swift was resourceful and got the job done.

In the early 1860s, army surgeon Joseph Howland Bill, MD, designed a pair of tong-like forceps for removing arrowheads. He studied over 150 cases of traumatic injuries inflicted by arrows. His first army assignment was at Fort Defiance, New Mexico Territory.

At the very heart of old letters, journals and military records lay flesh-and-blood human beings. To them, deep respect and humble appreciation is offered—for it was they who lived the stories. It was they who made possible this trip back through time via stories at the core of this book.

**FACTOID** Some Native American peoples traditionally treated an arrow wound by sucking it and filling it with pulverized peyote root, cleaning it several times and adding more peyote powder over the next few days, then finally covering the wound with pulverized lechuguilla root. Such plants were critical for treating the ills and injuries of Native peoples in the desert.

## Further Reading

Bill, "Forceps for the Extraction of Arrow-heads," *Medical Record 1876*, 245.
Centers for Disease Control. *"Table 15. Life Expectancy at Birth."*
Quebbeman, *Medicine in Territorial Arizona*, 4–5.
Smith, Thompson, Wooster and Pingenot, *Reminiscences of Maj. Gen. Zenas R. Bliss*, 56.

## CHAPTER 3

# BARROOM BRAWL, DEATH, HANGING

**A**lcohol undoubtedly inflamed tempers and exacerbated situations, sometimes leading to violence. One incident involving civilians and Eighth U.S. Infantry soldiers of Company G happened in 1860 on St. Patrick's Day—which was probably a popular day with soldiers. At that time, according to U.S. Census records, 47 percent of the soldiers at Fort Davis were Irish.

At Daniel Murphy's saloon just outside the Fort Davis army post, a fight broke out. A soldier was stabbed to death, presumably by the civilian bartender.

When the dead soldier's angry comrades—no doubt under the influence of alcohol—began to avenge the death of their fellow soldier, wild gunfire in the dark night led to yet another soldier being mortally wounded. The army surgeon's death record later noted the second man was "shot through the head by a drunken soldier and killed instantly."

With two soldiers dead—John Pratt and Michael Powers—a riot ensued. The panicked bartender, William Graham, feared for his life—and rightly so.

No local civil law enforcement existed at the time, so the garrison's officer of the day was summoned. He and a military guard persuaded the fear-stricken bartender to seek refuge in the guardhouse—also known as the post stockade or "jail" for protection.

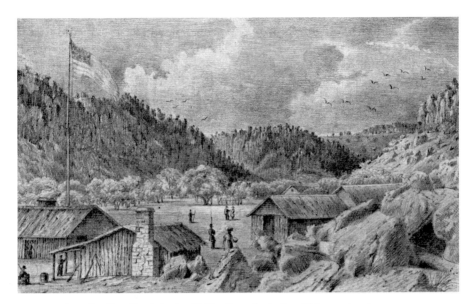

While stationed at Fort Davis in the 1850s, Captain Arthur T. Lee painted many scenes. This one shows the guardhouse (*foreground*). *Fort Davis NHS.*

That saved his life, but only temporarily. The next day or soon afterwards, a group of soldiers—with the aid of six sympathetic army jail guards—dragged the bartender to a tree and hanged him.

The U.S. Army's commander of the Department of Texas, Lieutenant Colonel Robert E. Lee, was determined to get to the bottom of this series of undisciplined actions. Lee, who was probably in San Antonio at the time, ordered a military investigation.

In solidarity with one another, however, the soldiers refused to identify those in the lynching party. Members of the jail guard who had let the prisoner be taken away were given stiff fines, plus sentences of eight to ten months of hard labor.

For trial, the army transported the presumed ringleaders to El Paso under heavy escort. The trial was dismissed for insufficient evidence.

**FACTOID** Since there are no photos of pre–Civil War Fort Davis, Captain Arthur T. Lee's works of art provide a lens through which to look back in time to the 1850s. Today, on exhibit panels near Hospital Canyon where the first Fort Davis was located, several of Lee's paintings help park visitors visualize what the first Fort Davis looked like. Lee and his wife, Margaret, had a total of five children, but only one of them survived childhood.

In the end, the army resolved the crime by dispersing members of Company G into other companies in the regiment. It was never discovered whether the bartender was guilty of the murder or had acted in self-defense. The guilty parties were never brought to trial.

## *Further Reading*

U.S. Census, 1860, Presidio County, Texas.
Wooster, *History of Fort Davis*, 141–42.

## CHAPTER 4

# DIPHTHERIA

## Strangling Angel of Death

**D**iphtheria was a frightening disease, though we hardly think about it nowadays—thanks to vaccines. In the nineteenth century, it was a major cause of death, especially among children.

In February 1881, diphtheria took the life of the young daughter of Fort Davis hospital steward L.H.L. Williamson and his wife. Born in New Mexico Territory in 1876, the little girl was named Centennia America, presumably to honor the nation's one hundredth birthday. When she succumbed to diphtheria, she was almost five years old—and was the Williamsons' only child. (There were no vaccines at the time, except for smallpox—which involved taking material from a blister of someone infected with cowpox and inoculating it into another person's skin, known as arm-to-arm inoculation.)

Sadly, although hospital stewards had access to the best medicine of the time, Williamson could not save his child from this dreaded disease. Young Centennia America was buried in the post cemetery. Later that year, the Williamsons left Fort Davis. Maybe the memories were overwhelming.

Diphtheria was called the Strangling Angel of Death because of the membrane that develops and blocks the airway, suffocating the victim. A few doctors used sharp instruments to poke a hole in the throat membrane and insert a tube to prevent suffocation. Then, if the immune system was strong enough, the child might survive. It was a form of

**FACTOID** The word *diphtheria* comes from the Greek *dipthera*, which means "leather." It refers to the thick, gray, leathery membrane that grows in the throat.

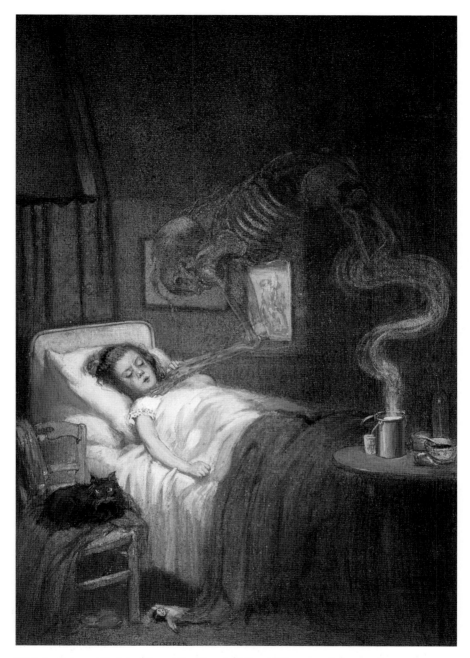

Diphtheria was called the "Strangling Angel of Death" because of the membrane that grew in the throat and blocked the victim's airway. *Richard Tennant Cooper, Wellcome Collection.*

tracheotomy and intubation—a rather drastic, traumatizing procedure for the child and parents.

Diphtheria was also called the Kiss of Death, and it sometimes killed adults. In 1878, Queen Victoria's thirty-five-year-old daughter, Princess Alice, died of diphtheria. Alice, her husband and their children fell ill with diphtheria, but only four-year-old Marie and then Alice died. A British medical journal warned that diphtheria could be spread even through the innocent kiss of a mother and child.

Not long after the deaths of Princess Alice in Germany and little Centennia America at Fort Davis, scientists in Europe were working diligently to isolate the diphtheria bacillus. By 1890, they had a genuine understanding of the disease. A diphtheria vaccine was developed in the 1920s and became commercially available in the 1940s.

Unfortunately, these advances in medicine did not help some of the people in Fort Davis when a diphtheria epidemic hit the town. It was the fall of 1891, only a few months after the army shut down the garrison. According to oral history and scanty documentation, the diphtheria epidemic in the town of Fort Davis resulted in twenty-one deaths.

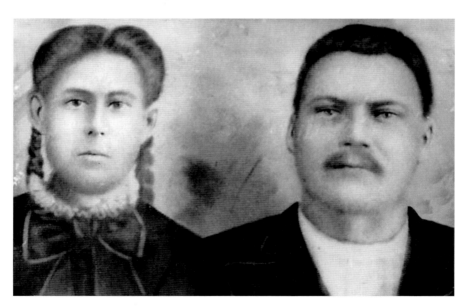

Concepcion and George Bentley buried all seven of their children due to a diphtheria epidemic that hit the town of Fort Davis in late 1891. *Fort Davis NHS.*

One family devastated by the 1891 diphtheria epidemic was that of George Bentley, a former Ninth Cavalry soldier who remained in Fort Davis after honorable discharge and worked for the army as a contractor. He and his wife, Concepcion, lost all seven of their children in less than three weeks' time and buried them in the town's Pioneer Cemetery. It is difficult to even contemplate such a tragedy.

After the dreadful event, Mr. and Mrs. Bentley had several more children—remarkable, considering Concepcion was about forty-four in 1891. (In the 1880 census, her age was recorded as thirty-three and George's as thirty-five.)

**FACTOID** Even Hippocrates knew of diphtheria over two thousand years ago. We now understand it is a bacterial infection, spread through the air via close contact with respiratory secretions. Children often contracted it from drinking cow's milk, which people in the nineteenth century did not know to heat or "pasteurize" to kill germs. The pasteurization process came from French scientist Louis Pasteur, whose medical discoveries in the 1860s and '70s provided support for the germ theory of disease—among the greatest breakthroughs in modern medicine.

According to family stories, George and Concepcion's strong faith is what got them through the loss of their seven children to diphtheria. They believed that God needed their children to be his angels. The Bentleys' second family consisted of three children—George Jr., Josephina and Lupe—who grew to adulthood, and their descendants live today in Fort Davis and elsewhere. Ah, the resilience of the human spirit!

## Further Reading

Cantwell (descendant of Bentleys), author interview, 2019.

Hardy, *The Epidemic Streets: Infectious Disease and the Rise of Preventive Medicine*, 82.

Jacobson and Nored, *Jeff Davis County, Texas*, 359.

Museum of Health Care at Kingston, "Diphtheria" (for Princess Alice information).

Rothstein, *American Physicians in the 19th Century*, 60, 272.

## CHAPTER 5

# NO PENSION FOR HER OWN WORK

Things can sure get convoluted when trying to get an army pension!
This story starts with a fifteen-year-old army laundress named Ellen Beck, who was part Cherokee. In 1874 at Fort Sill, Oklahoma Territory, she married a soldier, George Goldsby, whose military service dated to the Civil War. When they married, he served with the all-Black Tenth U.S. Cavalry.

Between 1878 and 1879, Sergeant Goldsby was involved in some ugly interracial incidents at Fort Concho. He organized Black soldiers in confronting racial violence. Then, to keep from being lynched in what was called "frontier justice," he deserted from the U.S. Army. He disappeared to build a new life in Kansas and changed his name—leaving behind Ellen and their four children. She struggled but continued to work as an army laundress.

Ten years later, Ellen married another soldier, William Lynch. They were married for twenty-seven years. After he died in 1916, Ellen applied for a widow's pension, but it was denied because she had never divorced Goldsby. She started signing her name as "Ellen Goldsby." Then, after George Goldsby died in 1922, she reapplied for a widow's pension—and it was granted, based on her 1874 marriage to George Goldsby.

Complicating Ellen's pension claim for her first husband's army service was the fact that George Goldsby—under the assumed name William Scott—had been married for forty years to his second wife, Effie Henshaw,

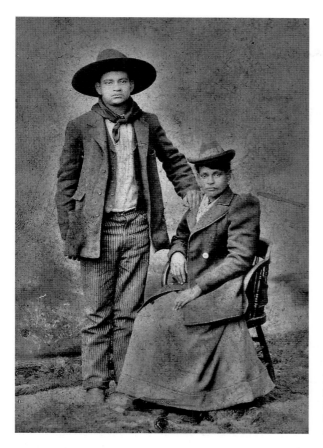

Ellen Beck Goldsby Lynch, shown here in 1896 with one of her sons. *From* Hell on the Border *by S.W. Harman, 1898.*

and they had six children. Effie tried to claim his pension for military service, but her claim was denied because there was no proof that George and Ellen had divorced.

Ellen lived for ten more years after her pension claim for George Goldsby's military service was granted, and she died in 1932 in Oklahoma at age seventy-three. In her pension claim, she stated that she had worked for the U.S. Army as what she called an "authenticated laundress" at multiple military posts, including Fort Concho in Texas and Fort Gibson in Oklahoma Territory.

This brings up the question: What about pensions for army women based on their own work?

The National Archives has on file almost 2,500 pension applications from women for their own service as nurses in the Civil War from 1861 to 1865. Not until 1892 did Congress sign into law the Army Nurses Pension Act (ANPA).

The ANPA entitled all women who had served as nurses in the Union army during the Civil War to a pension of twelve dollars per month—as long as they had served for six months and had been hired by a person authorized by the War Department to hire nurses.

This did not apply to Ellen Beck Goldsby Lynch because she was not a nurse—or a laundress—during the Civil War. She was a young child then.

Despite the fact that the ANPA law excluded army laundresses, scouts, cooks and Southern women, it was a huge achievement for women, made possible by years of work aided by the Women's Relief Corps and the Army Nurses' Association. It was also the first time the federal government recognized—and thus legitimized—women's service in the Civil War army.

This story reveals how slow America was to acknowledge nineteenth-century women's contributions to the military.

Over a twenty-five-year period after the Civil War, Congress passed about two hundred acts or laws that granted women pensions based on their own military service rather than that of a husband or son—but only if they had been single during their army service and then remained unmarried afterward.

Lawmakers apparently saw no need for a married woman to receive money in compensation for services that she rendered, risking her own health and life to do so.

## Further Reading

Leiker, "George Goldsby," 137–57.
Metheny, "For a Woman: The Fight for Civil War Army Nurses."

## CHAPTER 6

# QUANAH PARKER AND PEYOTE

## Indigenous Cactus Medicine

**P**eyote is a small, spineless cactus, but it can pack a wallop when ingested because of its narcotic content. The original Nahuatl root word, *peyōtl*, means "glistening." Indigenous peoples of the Americas are believed to have used peyote in healing and religious ceremonies for over five thousand years.

Quanah Parker, Comanche leader of the Quahadi band, was one of the notable figures who visited the army post of Fort Davis. He was the son of Comanche chief Peta Nocona and Cynthia Ann Parker—a White woman captured as a child in 1836 and raised by Comanches, who called her Naduah.

**FACTOID** Peyote cactus contains substances—especially mescaline, known for its hallucinogenic effects—that affect brain function and produce an altered state of consciousness. Peyote has been used for medicinal purposes to treat conditions such as cold, fever, asthma, diabetes, hysteria, toothache, blindness, rheumatism, breast pain, skin diseases and pain in childbirth.

In 1884, Quanah reportedly traveled south from his home in Oklahoma in search of peyote, since that plant did not exist in the area around Fort Sill where he lived. Others say he went to southwest Texas to search for roots of a "plant to counteract malaria," hoping to take the roots back home to cultivate new plants.

At Fort Davis, Quanah stayed briefly as a guest in the home of Captain Charles L. Cooper and his family. Cooper's teenage daughter Forrestine—called "Birdie"—recalled the visit in her memoirs.

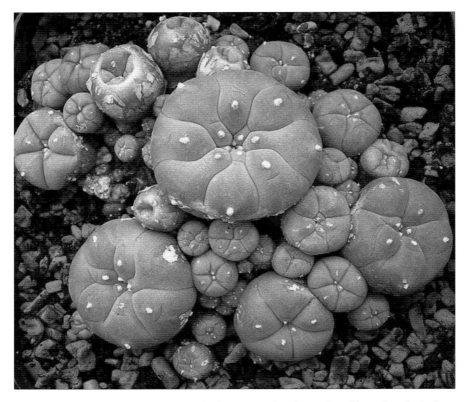

Peyote is an extremely slow-growing, spineless cactus. Specimens found in archaeological digs date back several thousand years or more. *Frank Vicentz, Wikimedia Commons.*

One of Quanah's traveling companions, George Fox of Philadelphia, suffered from tuberculosis and hoped drier climatic conditions in the West would help. Unfortunately, however, George died from the disease not long after his trip to Texas.

Lieutenant John Bigelow wrote in his journal that Quanah was traveling with two other "Indians" and that when the group departed Fort Davis on the cold, drizzly morning of December 10, 1884, Quanah was wearing a lieutenant's uniform. He was accompanied by Lieutenant Powhatan Clarke and six soldiers. Quanah had requested the army escort; perhaps it was felt he would be safer that way. After ten days in the field, Quanah and Fox again stayed with the Cooper family before returning to the Fort Sill reservation.

No one knows how many plant-collecting trips Quanah Parker made to west Texas and Mexico. Twentieth-century author Barry Scobee says Quanah stayed in town in Fort Davis at the Lempert Hotel, now the Veranda Historic Inn. Others say Quanah stayed at the Hotel Limpia.

**FACTOID** The Drug Enforcement Administration (DEA) lists peyote as a controlled substance, but many state and federal laws, like the American Indian Religious Freedom Act, protect peyote's harvest, cultivation and consumption by Native peoples for religious ceremonies.

So why peyote—if that is what Quanah was searching for? The story goes that Quanah had been gored by a bull or injured by buffalo hunters earlier in his life and that a Mexican *curandera* (Native healer) had treated him using peyote. After that, Quanah became involved in the Native American Church, which was a religious movement using peyote in its rituals.

In her memoirs, Birdie Cooper wrote that Quanah was a frequent guest in the Cooper home in the 1870s when her father was stationed at Fort Sill, Oklahoma. Quanah called her Cooper's Girl and liked to hear her play on the piano, which he called "thunder music."

## Further Reading

Bigelow, *Garrison Tangles in the Friendless Tenth*.

Fisher, "Forrestine Cooper Hooker [...] Notes on Army Life in the West, 1871–1876."

Hooker, *Child of the Fighting Tenth: On the Frontier with the Buffalo Soldiers*.

CHAPTER 7

# A YOUNG BOY LOSES HIS FATHER

T he coffin for Captain James Hill Patterson, Twenty-Fifth U.S. Infantry, cost nine dollars when he died at age thirty in 1873 at Fort Davis. The post quartermaster hired a carpenter to build it.

It must have been a very sad farewell. His wife, Elizabeth Vandegrift Patterson, was twenty-seven. His small son, John Love Patterson, called Johnny, would turn five years old the following week.

Captain Patterson had complained of vertigo, and the army surgeon admitted him to the hospital. He died two weeks later of what the army surgeon described as "Acute Articular Rheumatism complicated with Acute Pericarditis." It's not clear what his cause of death was. It was possibly an autoimmune disease—little understood in the nineteenth century.

Following is an excerpt from the post surgeon's death report, with a description of the elaborate military funeral procession to the post cemetery:

> *Died at 10:55 AM on Aug. 19 and buried the next day in the Post Cemetery with military ceremonies at 5 PM in the following order of procession—1st: Band, 2nd: Escort composed of D Company, 25th Infantry, Captain D.D. Van Valzah, Commanding, 3rd: Corpse and bearers, 4th: G Company 25th Infantry, 5th: Carriages, 6th: I Company, 9th Cavalry, 7th: C Company, 25th Infantry, 8th: Citizens, 9th: Officers of the Garrison in inverse order of rank. The attendance at his funeral manifested the esteem in which he was held by his brother officers, the troops, and citizens of Fort Davis.*

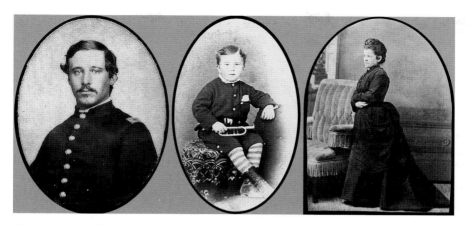

Captain James Hill Patterson; his wife, Elizabeth; and their son John Love. *Photos courtesy of John Patterson Lindley, Bradley, California.*

Not long afterwards, Captain Patterson's wife and son vacated their Fort Davis quarters on Officers' Row. They traveled east under army escort—starting out in a wagon and camping along the way, eventually arriving back home in Indiana. This was before the railroads came to west Texas.

Even as an old man, years later, Captain Patterson's son, Johnny, remembered details of that trip, which must have been quite an adventure for a five-year-old boy. He recalled that once, when he pulled a stick out of the campfire and waved it around, the soldiers reminded him they were trying to keep a low profile to not attract "Indians."

Five months after the funeral, the body of Captain Patterson was disinterred from Fort Davis at his parents' expense and shipped back to Indianapolis to be reinterred at Crown Hill Cemetery. There he was buried in the family plot next to his only other sibling—a sister, Eudora, who had died in childbirth two years earlier.

Elizabeth applied for—and was granted—a pension from the Department of the Interior's Bureau of Pensions. Her husband's military career had begun in 1862 during the Civil War. The amount of her widow's pension was twenty dollars per month, plus an additional two dollars for her child. She also taught piano lessons to help support herself and her son.

When Elizabeth remarried nine years later, in 1882, to another Civil War veteran, James Livingston Mitchell, her pension from Captain Patterson's service ceased, but that of their son John Love continued for a couple years, until his sixteenth birthday. Five years after Elizabeth remarried, during which time she gave birth to another son, Frank, she was again widowed. She lived for thirty more years and died in 1917 at age seventy-one.

The story was told to me by Captain Patterson's great-grandson over fifteen years ago as we sat on a bench at the Fort Davis Post Cemetery. How touching that this kind man, John Patterson Lindley, no longer young himself, traveled all the way from California to revisit the fort where his great-grandfather had served and died. He even got to sit in the shade of a small, gnarled tree at the old cemetery—where his great-grandfather, a handsome captain who served as company commander of his regiment, had originally been buried after his untimely death many, many years earlier.

## *Further Reading*

Lindley (great-grandson of Captain James H. Patterson), communication with author, 2002–present.

U.S. Army, Medical History of Posts and Records of Adjutant General's Office—Registers of the Sick and Wounded. Fort Davis NHS archival library.

## CHAPTER 8

# FRONTIER MILITARY WOMEN SOMETIMES TOOK MATTERS INTO THEIR OWN HANDS

S tories of army women, like the one in this chapter of Emma Beeks—and the abortion that ended up killing her—give insight into the private lives of women rarely discussed in old letters, journals or army records.

Before birth control was readily available, women sometimes took matters into their own hands to end unwanted pregnancies. Abortions were legal in the nineteenth century until 1873, as long as they were performed before "quickening" (when the mother can first feel movement in the womb)—but they were dangerous.

Information about abortion was available to women, whether they were educated or not. Even though some researchers believe abortion was more prevalent among middle- and upper-class women because they could better afford the costs of such a service, historian Darlis Miller wrote in 1986 that it is clear women of all classes underwent abortions. As she explained, the story of Emma Beeks at Fort Union, New Mexico Territory, in 1879 reveals that lower-class women, who did not have written traditions, nevertheless shared knowledge about abortions and helped one another when necessary.

Herbs known to cause abortion or miscarriage included wild tansy, ergot, aloes, savin, squill, nutmeg, saffron, mugwort, pennyroyal, snakeroot, motherwort, black cohosh, wild carrot, senna/black draught, common rue and cotton-root bark. Some could be violent purgatives. Even turpentine was

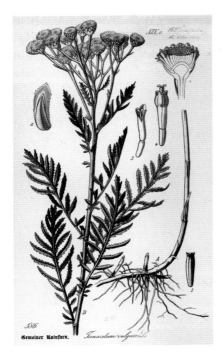

Tansy is a powerful and potentially dangerous herb in the aster family. It has long been used for various medical conditions. *Drawing by Otto Thomé, 1885; Wikimedia Commons.*

used, as well as oil of cedar, ergot of rye, mallow and motherwort. Sources indicate that Native Americans used the mistletoe plant or berries to bring on an abortion.

Army laundresses, female servants, midwives and officers' wives might have grown their own herbs or obtained them from other local knowledgeable sources, including Native healers (*curanderas*). Pills containing concoctions of herbs were available as over-the-counter patent medicine. Some were known as emmenagogues—to bring on monthly menstrual periods.

The death rate from abortion was as high as 30 percent—more than the death rate from childbirth, which certainly carried risk. To dilate the cervix in order to induce abortion or miscarriage, women used a variety of items—catheters, glass rods, candles, needles, spoons, sticks or knives.

Both oral traditions and written sources tell us that women helped each other with herbal medicine traditions handed down through generations.

Here's the story of one frontier officer's servant who took matters into her own hands—and lost the gamble. Emma Beeks was thirty-five years old when she died at Fort Union in March 1879. Cause of death was listed as "peritonitis and hemorrhage from criminal abortion."

Born in Georgia, Emma Beeks was single, Black and lived on laundresses' row. She worked as a servant in the home of the family of the post surgeon, Carlos Carvallo, MD. The abortion occurred when Dr. Carvallo was temporarily away from the post. Autopsy revealed that the wall of Beeks's vagina had been punctured by a sharp instrument. She died from loss of blood and infection.

A hospital matron/laundress named Margaret Berry testified at the trial that the dead woman had ingested a concoction of whiskey with wild tansy, a well-known abortifacient. Borax was also in the mixture, according to Dr.

**FACTOID** Army medical records in the nineteenth century generally documented treatment of enlisted men and officers—all male—not women (who were "civilians," even those who worked as laundresses or hospital matrons). It is unclear whether army doctors performed abortions, but at times, they likely did help women limit the size of their families. Listed on the *Standard Supply Table of the Medical Department of the U.S. Army, 1871*, from which doctors could order supplies, are ergot, aloes, squill and turpentine. These medications had varied medicinal uses.

ERGOT is derived from a fungus or mushroom. It has long been used to stop maternal bleeding after childbirth or to induce contractions to cause the fetus to be aborted.

SQUILL is from the bulbs of lily-like plants. It can induce vomiting; treat lung infections, bronchitis and whooping cough; serve as a heart tonic; relieve fluid retention; and cause abortion.

ALOES, taken from cactus-like plants, have been used in traditional medicines for thousands of years for burns, colitis, bleeding, seizures, hemorrhoids, osteoarthritis, eye conditions, as laxatives and to bring on menstrual periods.

Carvallo, who suspected that Berry had assisted with the abortion since she had previously been involved with other abortions. One man testified that Margaret Berry had performed an abortion on his wife—Berry's own daughter—and would do so whenever her daughter got pregnant.

At the time of her death, Emma Beeks had a sixteen-month-old son. Investigation into the case disclosed that less than a year before the abortion that killed her, Beeks had aborted another unwanted pregnancy.

Later, Dr. Carvallo proved that Margaret Berry—who also lived on laundresses' row—had pilfered some of the dead woman's clothing and created a ruckus among the laundresses. The army expelled Berry from the Fort Union garrison.

## Further Reading

Miller, "Foragers, Army Women, and Prostitutes," 155–56.
Mohr, *Abortion in America: Origins and Evolution of National Policy, 1800–1900*, 628.
Oliva, *Fort Union and the Frontier Army in the Southwest*, 628.

## CHAPTER 9

# TWO MORE WOMEN WHO TOOK
# MATTERS INTO THEIR OWN HANDS

A t Fort Buford, Northern Dakota Territory, in October 1878, an
army laundress named Margaret Littlejohn died from an abortion.
She was thirty-six.

Publicly, her death was listed as being due to complications from a
miscarriage, but official records say it was due to abortion. It is unknown
who performed the abortion—perhaps, on her own, Margaret concocted
and drank the potion that killed her.

Margaret was married to a soldier, Private Amos W. Littlejohn, who had
started his military service during the Civil War with the Indiana Infantry.
They had married in 1865 in Indiana. At the time of her death, she and
Amos had three daughters: Violet, Lillie and Vesta Martha.

Apparently, the soldiers had high regard for their laundress, for when
Margaret died they erected a gravestone for her. She was buried in the Fort
Buford Post Cemetery but later reinterred at Custer National Cemetery in
Montana after Fort Buford closed in 1895.

Census records reveal that Margaret was herself the oldest of ten
children of Mary and Daniel Caton, so she obviously came from a prolific
family. Perhaps Margaret, like many women then, found ways to limit the
size of her family.

Another story of terminated pregnancy took place at Fort Garland,
Colorado, in 1876. An officer's wife from New York named Emma Jane—
the nineteen-year-old wife of Lieutenant John Conline—traveled to the

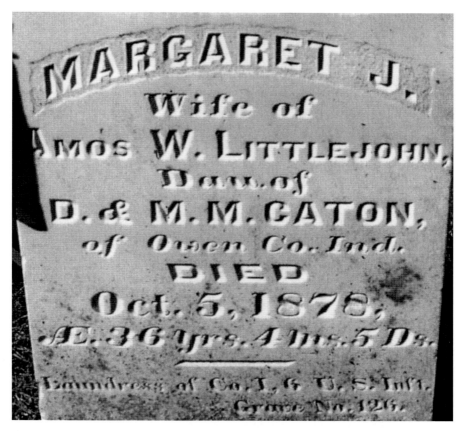

Margaret Littlejohn's gravestone today at Custer National Cemetery. *Author's collection.*

nearby town of La Veta for an abortion. There, she complained that the army doctors at the fort had refused to perform the abortion. The couple had a one-year-old daughter, Viola.

After Emma returned to the garrison and resumed life, rumors abounded about her behavior. She was accused of spreading malicious gossip, using "unladylike and violent language," speaking openly of having an abortion, frequently spending time at the laundresses' quarters, talking to soldiers on guard duty, appearing in a partial state of nudity at times and chasing one laundress with a gun. Any of these actions would have been considered conduct unbecoming an officer's wife and a Victorian lady, but combined, it became clear that Emma had become a spectacle, a nuisance and an embarrassment.

Medical practitioners at the time tended to diagnose a woman's unusual behavior as being caused by "emotional fits of insanity." Thus, in 1877, the post commander ordered Emma to leave Fort Garland on grounds that she was "insane" and was disturbing "the peace and order" of the garrison. Her husband, after first resisting the charge and even enduring arrest for forty days while he appealed the order to higher authority, finally agreed to escort his wife back to New York, and then he returned to Fort Garland.

Their marriage ended in divorce two years later. Emma had been fifteen when she married twenty-five-year-old John Conline, an 1870 West Point graduate from Vermont. After the divorce, Lieutenant Conline continued his career at other military posts. There's no report telling what happened to Emma or their daughter, Viola.

**FACTOID** Army medical report describing Margaret Littlejohn's death: "October 6, 1878 Mrs. Littlejohn, a laundress of Co. I, 6th Infantry, died in the Post Hospital at 8 o'clock last evening, after a sickness of 19 months. Her death resulted from a complication of maladies the remote cause however being an abortion in the 3rd month followed by later efluxion and metritis [inflammation of uterine wall]. Subsequently she suffered with cystitis, pelvic cellulitis, obstinate and uncontrollable vomiting, uterine hyperplasia [enlargement]... constipation, and finally pelvis peritonitis, and an aggravation of the cellulites. Death occurred by asthenia [extreme weakness] and by gradual diminution of the vital forces. Autopsy: 16 hours after death."

## Further Reading

Harvey, *Fort Buford Medical Report*, 1878.
Lawrence, *Soap Suds Row: Bold Lives of Army Laundresses, 1820–1878*, 77.
Medical History of Fort Buford, Dakota Territory.
Sauerwein, communication with author.
Tavernier, "Major John Conline, 1846–1916."

# CHAPTER 10

# MAGIC LANTERNS AND PHOTOGRAPHY

Dr. John Vance Lauderdale, post surgeon at Fort Davis from 1888 to 1890, had a most inquiring mind. He was an avid reader of medical journals and newspapers. Always interested in experimenting with new mechanical things, he rigged up a telephone line from his home to the post hospital for calling his hospital steward. He also loved dabbling with the equipment that made ice for the post hospital to treat fever.

An amateur photographer as well, Dr. Lauderdale had some elaborate camera equipment. Plus, he was always eager for news of the latest in photography, such as what Eastman Kodak was doing in camera development.

Dr. Lauderdale was fifty-five when the army moved him and his family to Fort Davis after a tour of duty at Fort Clark. His wife, Josephine "Joe" Lane Lauderdale, was thirty-six and their toddler, Marjorie, almost two. It was not always an easy life—three years before, they had buried their first child, a daughter, at not quite three weeks old.

Within a few months of their arrival at Fort Davis, Dr. Lauderdale had rigged up a darkroom in the post hospital, where he developed his own photos on glass plates. Soon he was showing "magic lantern" slideshows for the Fort Davis troops and people of the garrison, who were no doubt

**FACTOID** On November 1, 1888, Dr. Lauderdale wrote in his journal: "The Eastmans are in the market with a small camera that has a roll of paper which will take one hundred views by the instantaneous method without changing the roll. The Kodak Camera it is called."

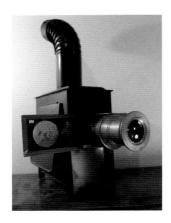

A magic lantern required "limelight" to project images of glass slides. It was an early version of modern slide projectors. *Andrei Niemimaki, Wikimedia Commons.*

eager for such entertainment—except near payday, as he noted in his journal.

Electricity had not yet come to Fort Davis, so the illumination for the magic lantern was provided by "limelight." The process: Vent some hydrogen gas and oxygen gas onto limestone. Then light the gases, which turn incandescent and create a strong light—the source of illumination in the magic lantern. (The saying "in the limelight" comes from the bright light generated by this technique.) Dr. Lauderdale had to produce his own oxygen and hydrogen gas.

During his lantern exhibitions, he showed commercially produced travel slides of Ireland, Scotland, Switzerland, America, Mexico, Pueblo villages and more—as he described in his journal, "Western scenery along the line of the Rocky Mountains as far north as the Yellow Stone Park."

Dr. Lauderdale faithfully kept a journal, and in it he mentioned conducting lantern entertainments in "the Hall." This was possibly a place in an unoccupied barracks, which army records show had a theater, barber shop and reading room.

On December 14, 1889, he wrote:

> *We prepared the hydrogen this morning for the lime light, and all the improvised apparatus worked well....This evening at 7.o clock. My* [hospital] *Steward who is handy at a good many things was equal to the task of managing the light, so that I could devote my attention to the lecture. The room was well filled with soldiers and their friends. Marjorie and her Mexican maid were there....The pictures showed well, and we had got through with upwards of 60 of the Mexican views when the hydrogen gave out....*

At Marjorie's third birthday party, Dr. Lauderdale took a photo indoors using his flash magnesium lamp—a marvel on the frontier. At the time, the average person could not afford to own a camera. In 1888, when the first Kodak cameras came on the market, such a camera cost twenty-five dollars, which included a leather carrying case. It came from the factory loaded with a roll of film that took one hundred exposures. Then the camera was shipped back to New York, where for ten dollars the pictures were developed, a new roll of film was loaded and the camera was returned to the owner. Amateur photographers who didn't want to mess with chemicals in a darkroom loved it.

What fun for young Marjorie to have a father who loved to tinker with scientific things. When she was three and a half, in March 1890, he penned:

> *Marjorie and I made hydrogen...for the lantern entertainment this evening. I had a quantity of gas left after filling the bag, and with this I made soap bubbles and amused the child by letting her see bubbles that would float upward to the ceiling instead of settling down to the floor as bubbles filled with air from the lungs do. I had one of the men place a lighted candle near these little balloons, but at a safe distance from the pipes, and let M. see the explosion. This she was a little startled at, and made her way a safe distance away from the pyrotechnics.*

Dr. Lauderdale's intellectual inquisitiveness seemed to drive everything he did. He also revealed a dry sense of humor: his wife gave birth at home on Thanksgiving Day 1889 to their son Vance. A week later, the doctor mentioned the baby drinking condensed milk out of a bottle with a long tube attached because Vance "refused to take any nourishment from maternal sources, which do not afford quite enough for his babyship."

Lauderdale's letters, journals and original photographic glass plates—accomplished when he was stationed at army posts throughout the West—provide insight into life on the frontier. Modern-day researchers are thankful he took pains to document everyday life in detail at a time when very few people could afford a camera. Among other things, his photos of Native Americans in the West reveal rich detail. His glass plates and journals are preserved today at Yale University's Beinecke Library. Although his beloved wife died at sixty-one, the good doctor lived to be ninety-eight.

**FACTOID** Dr. Lauderdale enjoyed meeting other camera owners. On February 8, 1889, he journaled: "A good many ladies are devoted to photography. Mrs Bowen [an officer's wife] showed some little gems of the art made by a Phila. lady with the Eastman Kodak camera which is so popular just now with every body who enjoy taking pictures and do not develop them." On April 1, 1889: "This afternoon Lieut DeFrees has been showing me some new things in photography viz exposing and developing the new flexible film (celluloid) plates—the article which is to supercede glass dry plates."

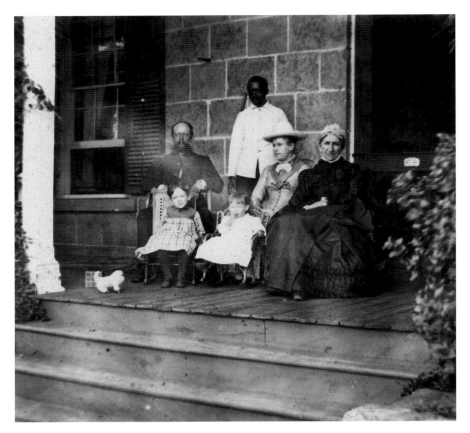

Dr. J.V. Lauderdale; his wife, Josephine; and their children Marjorie and Vance at home on Officers' Row, Fort Davis. House servant David Moore is standing; a guest is at right. *Lauderdale, Yale University, Beinecke Library.*

## *Further Reading*

Fort Davis National Historic Site archival library.
Greene, *Historic Resource Study: Fort Davis.*
Lauderdale, "Letterbooks, 1885–1892, Vols. 8–9."

## CHAPTER 11

# THE RUNS

## Diarrhea but No Issue of the Tissue (TP)

Diarrhea is mostly an inconvenience nowadays, but it was a killer in the nineteenth century. How did people try to treat diarrhea or dysentery when it commonly killed people?

Army medical records show that in the 1870s and 1880s, soldiers suffered and even died from dysentery—a water-borne disease. Soldiers and civilians alike drank untreated water right out of creeks and rivers.

In April 1884, the army at Fort Davis installed a new water system. High on the hillside, soldiers built a huge water tank—and then, two years later, another water tank—of cypress wood. Each tank held thirty-two thousand gallons of water, pumped uphill by a steam-driven pump from Limpia Creek where the water table was only three feet below the surface.

There was no treatment system at Fort Davis, however. Water pumped from the creek up to the tanks then flowed in pipes down to locations around the fort. Periodically, the tanks had to be cleaned out. Post surgeon Dr. William Gardner noted tadpoles in the water tanks during warm weather and forbade the water's use for anything but laundry. In 1886, he

**FACTOID** Dr. John Snow in London was one of the first people to start figuring it out—he traced cholera to a public water pump in the town square in 1854. At the time, the world was facing a cholera pandemic. Instead of blaming cholera on "miasma" (bad air), Dr. Snow's work pointed to water contaminated by London's sewage. He removed the handle of a public water pump so people could no longer drink the sewage-infected water—and cases of cholera subsided.

FACTOID In May 1888, Fort Davis post surgeon Dr. John Lauderdale recommended boiling and filtering the drinking water—as he noticed pollution near the well from cattle, goats, sheep and dead frogs.

ordered all water used at the hospital to be boiled and filtered, and he recommended that everyone at the post do the same. Dutifully, he sent water samples off to Washington to be analyzed—but reports at the time revealed only chemical content, not bacteria.

How did they treat "the runs" that people got from animals defecating at the water source? Opium was one of the most common drugs. Ipecac, too. A popular over-the-counter medicine was Dover's (or Dover) Powder—a combination of opium and ipecac.

To have on hand at the hospital dispensary, post surgeons could order eight-ounce bottles of powdered opium, eight-ounce bottles of powdered ipecac and sixteen-ounce bottles of Dover's Powder, as listed in the *Standard Supply Table of the Medical Department of the U.S. Army.* (This was the official list of drugs, medical supplies and equipment available to army doctors.)

Other diarrhea remedies included quinine, alum, iron, arsenic, calomel/mercury, sulphate of copper, acetate of lead, nitrate of silver, mineral acids, saline purgatives and nux vomica/strychnine.

Imagine having diarrhea without today's luxuries: toilet paper, bathrooms inside our heated or air-conditioned homes and a porcelain toilet that uses water to flush away waste into a sewer system. Conveniences that we take for granted did not exist at frontier military posts.

Step back in time and imagine a soldier suffering from diarrhea. The latrine he goes into is dark, smelly, cold in winter, hot in summer and might be harboring black widow spiders. His gut hurts, and as he sits there moaning in pain and passing watery or bloody stools, he doesn't have anything to wipe with. The army did not issue toilet paper. Quartermaster supply lists had writing paper and brown packaging paper, but no such thing as toilet paper or water closet paper.

In 1883, the U.S. Patent Office granted a patent for roll-based TP dispensers. Still,

FACTOID Privies/outhouses/latrines were part of the way diseases spread. A hygienic innovation from Europe in the 1860s–70s was the "earth closet." Fort Davis had at least one "earth closet," built in 1889 near the post hospital. It was outdoors—but instead of a hole in the ground, it had a big, deep wooden drawer or container filled with earth or sand, located under the toilet seat, which could be emptied when it filled with human waste. (Like today's litter boxes for cats.) By comparison, a toilet that flushed with water was called a "water closet."

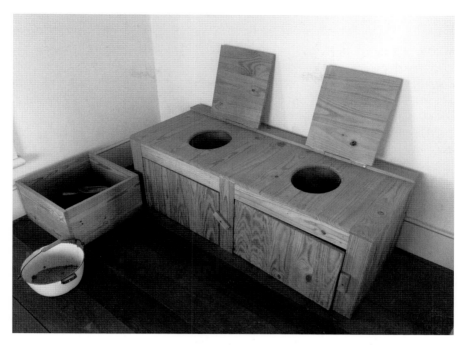

Earth closet inside Fort Concho post hospital. One of the two boxes has been removed from under the "toilet" seats and is visible at left. *Photo by author.*

frontier army posts did not boast such luxuries. Around 1890, the first perforated rolls of toilet paper were introduced.

It wasn't until 1893 that the U.S. War Department—for the first time—recognized toilet paper. General Order 56 authorized its purchase out of company funds.

Finally, in 1901, U.S. Army regulations institutionalized "issue of the tissue." It wasn't until 1930, however, that toilet paper was advertised as being "splinter free."

So, what did people long ago use for TP? If you imagine them using old newspaper or pages torn from catalogs, remember: random paper products were not plentiful at a time when many people were illiterate. What likely sufficed for most people were ordinary things like hay, rags, moss, grass, corncobs, seashells, animal fur, wood shavings and soft leaves. In certain countries, people used a spatula made of bamboo with the end wrapped in cloth. Some early cultures used a communal sponge on a stick. Others used pieces of pottery with names of enemies inscribed on them, then rinsed with water or snow.

**FACTOID** In America, toilet paper didn't emerge until 1857. A man in New York City named Joseph Gayetty first introduced TP. It was "medicated paper" infused with aloe and was not on rolls. Instead, it came in packages of flat sheets and was marketed as "the greatest necessity of the age." Cost for one thousand flat pieces was $1, and each sheet was marked with his name. Gayetty's advertisement warned against using regular printed paper or writing paper, which contained acids and other "fearful poisons." Ah, what tender considerations!

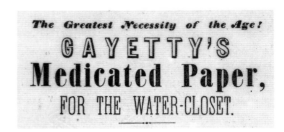

Gayetty's Medicated Paper for the Water-Closet—early toilet paper! Advertised in New York City, 1857. *Library of Congress.*

What *did* people use? Well, we can only guess—because such "unspeakable" things are not often mentioned in letters and journals. When nature calls, you find a way!

## *Further Reading*

Greene, *Historic Resource Study: Fort Davis*, 254–62.

Lauderdale, "Letterbooks, 1885–1892, Vols. 8–9."

U.S. War Department, *Standard Supply Table of the Medical Department of the United States Army, 1883*, 8, 12.

## CHAPTER 12

# IN THE LINE OF DUTY

## Baseball Injuries

In the early 1880s, the U.S. Army endorsed baseball as America's national pastime. Soldiers at frontier forts adopted the game with eagerness, and the military establishment embraced it as well. The sport offered wholesome, healthy entertainment, as well as a reprieve from soldiers' monotonous routine.

Equipment and rules varied from baseball today. Balls were softer, so long-distance hits were rare. Players used bare hands instead of leather gloves, making fingers vulnerable to injury. At bat, the player could call for a "high ball" or "low ball." Six balls gave the player a walk.

Sometimes, Fort Davis soldiers played a team of townspeople or a team of soldiers from a nearby sub-post such as Camp Peña Colorado near Marathon (about sixty miles away—a very long trip on a horse or in a wagon). In his journals, Fort Davis post surgeon Dr. John Lauderdale mentioned a game on February 22, 1889, between soldiers from Camp Peña Colorado and the "Fort Davis Club." It was a Friday and Washington's birthday—a national holiday beginning in 1885.

**FACTOID** On September 10, 1888, Dr. Lauderdale performed a partial finger amputation on a Fort Davis soldier, Private Henry Daven, Fifth U.S. Infantry. He was twenty-seven. *Register of the Sick and Wounded* says it was a severe lacerated wound of the second finger on the left hand, having been struck by a baseball. He amputated the top joint, using antiseptic precautions and injecting 4 percent cocaine solution at the site. The injury was considered "in the line of duty." On September 27, Daven was returned to duty, "cured."

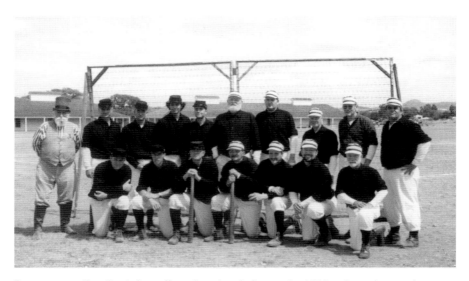

Reenactors at Fort Davis face off to play a baseball game by 1880s rules, using no gloves and wearing wool shirts and cotton long underwear. *Fort Davis NHS.*

As soon as baseball was introduced at Fort Davis in 1884, the post surgeon began reporting baseball injuries. In the next five years, medical records show there were at least fifteen such injuries treated at the hospital: fractures, lacerations, eye injuries, as well as sprains to hands, knees, hips, ankles and fingers.

It is easy to imagine how injuries happened to hands and fingers. No gloves for players except the catcher, who might wear a simple leather glove with the fingertips cut off and an opening in the back to admit air. In the mid-1870s, players who first started wearing gloves to protect their hands in places like Chicago and Boston were ridiculed for being weak.

At Fort Davis, two baseball injuries resulted in finger amputations. Such baseball-related injuries were considered to be "in the line of duty" and were notated as such in the hospital register, showing the official sanction of the sport.

Some troopers took great pride in their baseball teams and raised money to purchase uniforms and equipment. At Fort Davis in 1885, when Lieutenant John Bigelow ordered baseballs from Chicago for his troop of Tenth Cavalrymen, they already had bats and bases.

One baseball-related incident that occurred off the field involved two soldiers' wives feuding at Fort Keogh, Montana, in the 1890s. One woman

**FACTOID** Albert G. Spalding said: "The first glove I ever saw on the hand of a ball player in a game was worn by Charles C. Waite, in Boston, in 1875... playing at first base. The glove worn by him was of flesh color, with a large, round opening in the back." But that was back East, and such equipment was slow getting to the frontier—especially for soldiers who had to buy their own.

threatened the other with a baseball bat for burning trash too near her clean laundry drying on the clothesline. To resolve the issue, the officer of the day—responsible for maintaining order at the garrison—directed an off-duty soldier to "walk post" between the two women's quarters. By doing so, he managed to keep the peace and prevent what might have become a medical emergency. Soon, the women forgot their squabbles with each other and took their anger out on the officer. Problem solved.

Despite the popularity of the sport, baseball-related injuries were not always deemed to be "in the line of duty." Private George Turner was treated at the Fort Davis post hospital for brain concussion on December 22, 1882, after being clobbered by a comrade with a baseball bat. Whether this incident was malicious or accidental may never be known, but the surgeon's notation about the mishap was, "Not in the line of duty."

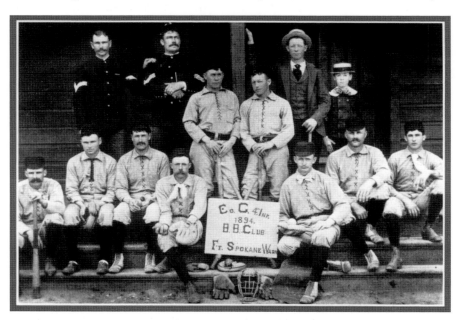

Baseball team at Fort Spokane, Washington, 1894. *Fort Davis NHS.*

*REPRINT OF*
*JULY 4, 1890 PROGRAM*

# GRAND FOURTH OF JULY CELEBRATION!

## AT FT. DAVIS, TEX.

❋ Lemonade, Coffee and Sandwiches Free. ❋

=10 A. M.=

## BASE BALL MATCH,

Old Nine Vs. Twenty-Third Infantry.
$9.00 Prize.

## LUNCH AT 12 M. AT THE PUMP HOUSE.

=COMMENCING AT 1 P. M.=

No. 1. Race for Boys, 10 yrs. and under, 60 yds. First Prize $1, Second Prize 50cts., Third Prize 25cts.

2. Race for Boys, 12 yrs. and under, 60 yds. First Prize $1, Second Prize 50cts., Third Prize 25cts.

3. Race for Boys, 15 yrs. and under, First Prize $1, Second Prize 50cts., Third Prize 25cts.

4. Potato race for girls, 12 Potatoes 1 yard apart. First Prize $1, Second Prize 50cts., Third Prize 25cts.

5. 100 yd. Dash, Open to All. First Prize $2, Second Prize $1.

6. Three Leg Race, 60 yards. Open to All. First Prize $2, Second Prize $1.

7. Throwing Base Ball. Three yards Run to Scratch. Prize $1.

8. High Jump. June Century for Rules. First Prize $2.

9. Running Broad Jump. June Century for Rules. First Prize $1.

10. Hurdle Race, 300 yards. Nine 2½ foot Hurdles. First Prize $5 Second Prize $1.

11. Sack Race, 40 yds. Open to All. First Prize $1, Second 50cts., Third Prize 25cts.

12. Wheel Barrow Race. Open to All. 40 yards. First Prize $5, Second Prize $2.

13. Burro Slow Race. Open to All. Once Around Parade Ground. First Prize $5, Second Prize $2.

14. Tug of War. Soldiers against Civilians. Twelve men to a side on bare ground. Prize $12.

15. Putting 12 pound shot. June Century for rules. Prize $3.

16. Putting 14 pound hammer. June Century for rules. Prize $3.

17. Long Foot Race, Once Around Parade Ground, Open to All. First Prize $10, Second Prize $2.50, Third Prize $1.

18. Catching Greased Pig. Prize "The Pig."

19. Fast Burro Race, Once around the Parade Ground. First Prize $5, Second Prize $2.

20. Pony Race, 14 hand high and under. 400 yards straight away. Mr. Dan Knight's Fast Horse ruled out. First Prize $25, Second Prize $5.

JUDGES WITH FULL POWER OF HORSE AND BURRO RACES—LIEUT. C. R. EDWBRDS and MR, H. M. PATTERSON.

JUDGES OF ALL FOOT RACES—LIEUT. J. L. T. PARTELLO and MR. S. A. THOMPSON.

JUDGES OF PUTTING SHOT, HAMMER, THROWING BASE BALL AND ALL JUMPING—LIEUT. W. H. C. BOWEN and MR. G. W. GLEIM.

JUDGE OF TUG OF WAR—COL. COCHRAN.

### By Order of Committee.

Printed flyer for Fourth of July celebration, 1890, at the Fort Davis garrison. *Fort Davis NHS.*

What a day it was at Fort Davis in 1890. July 4 was on a Friday, so everyone was, no doubt, ready to start celebrating. The main event was the baseball match at ten o'clock between teams Old Nine and the Twenty-Third Infantry—the prize: nine dollars. There was free lemonade, coffee and sandwiches. Lunch was at noon at the pump house along Limpia Creek. Games commenced at one o'clock: tug-of-war (twelve soldiers vs. twelve civilians), putting a twelve-pound shot or fourteen-pound hammer, wheelbarrow race, three-legged race, high jump, three-hundred-yard hurdle race, races for boys (by age group), potato race for girls, sack race, pony race (prize $25, but "Mr. Dan Knight's fast horse ruled out"), running broad jump, throwing baseball, slow burro race, race, fast burro race and catching a greased pig—in which the prize was the pig! Other prizes ranged from 25¢ to $10. What fun!

**FACTOID** As popular as baseball was at frontier army posts, at least one person felt it was sacrilegious to play baseball on Sundays. Fort Davis post surgeon John V. Lauderdale wrote this about a game in Marfa on Sunday, November 11, 1888: "Our unsanctified Commanding Officer and his 'satellite' the Post Adjutant left the Post (with their elder sons) at an early hour this morning, to witness a Baseball match at Marfa. Men with such principles are a disgrace to the Army as well as of no credit to the community."

## Further Reading

Barthelmess, *Photographer on an Army Mule*, 94–95.
Bigelow, *Garrison Tangles*, 33.
Bluthardt, "Baseball on the Military Frontier," 20–21.
EyeWitness to History.com, "Baseball Glove Comes to Baseball, 1875."
Lauderdale, "Letterbooks, 1885–1892, Vols. 8–9."
Stallard, *Glittering Misery: Dependents of the Indian Fighting Army*, 69.
Wooster, *History of Fort Davis*, 353.

## CHAPTER 13

# NOT IN THE LINE OF DUTY:
# MAN BITE

I njuries to soldiers were not always considered "in the line of duty." Violence was part of life at frontier army posts. Old medical records reveal countless fights and drunken brawls resulting in soldiers needing the attention of army doctors because of cuts and contusions of the face or scalp, fractures of the leg or hand—or worse. Usually, after these entries in the medical reports, the surgeon notated that the injury was "not in the line of duty."

"Man bite" occasionally shows up in the army medical records. One soldier was treated at the Fort Davis post hospital for "man bite to the lower lip, received while fighting."

A bloody "man bite" story happened in 1882 at Fort Davis when two soldiers got into a brawl and one man bit off the ear of the other soldier. On New Year's Day, Private James Henry lost his left ear in a fight with a comrade. This "man bite" tale is reminiscent of the June 1997 boxing match when Mike Tyson bit a chunk out of Evander Holyfield's right ear. As they say, there's nothing new under the sun.

Not infrequently, the Fort Davis surgeon wrote in the medical records that a soldier who was intoxicated when injured "did not remember how it happened."

On one such occasion, a trooper cut another soldier with a bottle. Another soldier fell while drunk and hurt himself. In a different incident, an innocent bystander was struck in the temple and injured by a rock thrown by one of the fighting parties—not considered official injuries "in the line of duty."

*Further Reading*

U.S. Army, Registers of the Sick and Wounded.

## CHAPTER 14

# WHO WILL PAY FOR DECEASED FRONTIER ARMY DOCTOR'S CASKET?

**D**eath came to army physicians too, for they were exposed to the same diseases and illnesses as soldiers.

In August 1885, while on active duty at Fort Concho, Texas, Dr. Samuel Moore Finley died of "acute peritonitis from the effect of renal calculus," leaving behind his wife and six-week-old baby. He was forty-three.

Finley, born in Pennsylvania, was an army contract surgeon or acting assistant surgeon—a civilian physician on temporary agreement or "contract" with the army, as opposed to doctors who were members of the U.S. Army Medical Department and had commissions as officers in the army. He had also been held as a prisoner of war (POW) by the Confederates during the Civil War. He then served for ten years as an army contract surgeon, no doubt hoping a vacancy would open up for him to become a regular medical officer in the army—although in the mid-1880s, when he died, Congress was cutting the Army Medical Department budget.

After Dr. Finley died, the Fort Concho post quartermaster put his body in a government burial casket and then asked the army to pay for it, stating the widow was "ill-able financially to stand the expense of the burial."

**FACTOID** U.S. Army regulations of 1881 stated that contract surgeons were paid a fixed amount of $100 to $125 per month. By comparison, commissioned medical officers received $133 to $208 per month depending on rank; salary increased with rank and tenure. Promotion was slow. It took Dr. Daniel Appel nineteen years and Dr. John V. Lauderdale twenty-one years to increase in rank from lieutenant to captain to major.

FRONTIER MEDICINE AT FORT DAVIS AND OTHER ARMY POSTS

**FACTOID** Some U.S. Army surgeons who served at Fort Davis and elsewhere and who died young by today's standards:

Dr. Paul Clendenin died at age thirty-nine from yellow fever in Cuba in 1899, during the Spanish American War.

Dr. Andrew Jackson Foard died in his forties of consumption (pulmonary TB) in 1868.

Dr. Albert Myer died at age fifty-two of Bright's Disease (a kidney condition now known as nephritis) in Buffalo, New York, in 1880. He is known as the "Father of the U.S. Army Signal Corps."

Dr. DeWitt Clinton Peters died at age forty-seven of phthisis pulmonalis (TB) in 1876 in Brooklyn after retiring less than five months earlier. Family history says he and his wife, Emily, were at Ford's Theater the night Lincoln was shot.

Dr. Daniel Weisel died at age fifty after falling sick on a march with troops in 1888 in Fort Sill, Indian Territory.

Ordinarily, the army did not pay for officers' funeral expenses, but the quartermaster mailed a letter requesting reimbursement for Dr. Finley's coffin. It went through the chain of command and ten endorsements all the way to the office of the surgeon general, who finally agreed the army would cover the expense.

One might wonder about the quartermaster's request for government reimbursement for a contract surgeon. If enlisted men, whose salary was between thirteen and twenty-three dollars per month, died on active duty, they were buried at the government's expense.

Dr. John Frazer Boughter, another army contract surgeon, died of consumption (TB) on January 16, 1876, while traveling with the army through Texas. He was buried at Fort Davis. The army was relocating Dr. Boughter to the lower Rio Grande in Texas for reasons of health. He was accompanying troops of the Eighth U.S. Cavalry from New Mexico to Fort Clark. When Boughter joined the battalion at Fort Bliss he was very ill. Shortly after they departed Fort Quitman, he died in an army ambulance in the arms of another contract surgeon, Dr. John Speed McLain. Apparently, the issue of payment for his casket at Fort Davis did not arise.

## *Further Reading*

Hume, *Ornithologists of the U.S. Army Medical Corps*, 134, 137–49.

Parker, *Records of the Association of Acting Assistant Surgeons of the United States Army* [1891], 65.

Smith, Thompson, Wooster and Pingenot, *Reminiscences of Major General Zenas R. Bliss*, 127.

U.S. War Department, *Regulations of the Army* [1881], article XII, paragraphs 122–23.

# CHAPTER 15

# SOLDIER BURIED HEADLESS

Early one afternoon in June 1878 at Fort Davis, Corporal Richard Robinson was shot in the head while asleep in his bunk. He was thirty-one and single. The crime was committed by Sergeant Moses Marshall. This was not an interracial crime; both soldiers were Black.

Dr. Ezra Woodruff, post surgeon, cleaned up the shattered skull, wired the pieces back together and shipped the skull off to Washington, D.C. It went to the Army Medical Museum, established for study as a research and teaching tool. The skull now sits in storage at the National Museum of Health and Medicine in Silver Spring, Maryland, near Washington, D.C.

The trial following the murder of Corporal Robinson was brief. Witnesses testified that alcohol was involved, that the two men were heard arguing before the incident and that the dead man had made disparaging remarks about Marshall's mother.

The civil court was composed of seven White men, who sentenced Marshall to serve ninety-nine years in prison. They sent him to the Texas State Penitentiary at Huntsville, which had been racially integrated just a few years earlier to include Blacks. Over four years later, he was transferred to the Texas State Penitentiary at Rusk.

**FACTOID** The official medical record of Corporal Robinson's death: "Shot through the head while sound asleep in his bed in the barracks & instantly murdered by Sergeant Moses Marshall of the same company. He was a good & faithful soldier—very popular in the command. This horrible death was lamented by all.... Buried the next day with the sacred and proud honors of religious and military ceremony in grave 56."

One wonders about the conditions at the Texas State Penitentiary in the 1880s and '90s. Discipline was reportedly harsh. Convicts performed physical labor, and prison guards were allowed to whip prisoners for poor daily work performance. Moses Marshall survived fourteen years in prison and died in September 1892 from "uraemia resulting from urethral stricture and subsequent surgical operation of external urethrotomy." In short, kidney failure—no doubt very painful. Although anesthesia was available at the time, this was before antibiotics for infection. In 1892, surgery on the urethra and its aftermath must have been excruciating.

Meanwhile, what happened to Corporal Robinson's body? Buried headless at Fort Davis in the West Cañon Post Cemetery, the body was not exhumed and moved with its marker in 1892 to the San Antonio National Cemetery like the bodies of other soldiers who died at Fort Davis. Robinson's name does not appear on the list of those disinterred, and nobody alive today knows why.

Whatever the reason, Robinson's bones remain at Fort Davis—somewhere. Only his skull, in museum storage, tells the gruesome story. In recent years, at least one modern-day park ranger avoided walking through the area south of the hospital where the 1878 West Cañon Post Cemetery was located. The ranger respectfully wanted to avoid crossing paths with the spirit of Corporal Richard Robinson.

**FACTOID** Beginning in 1862, Surgeon General William Hammond directed army physicians to send to the new Army Medical Museum in Washington, D.C., any body parts taken during autopsies or surgeries that might be instructive—e.g., a heart or lungs (such wet specimens were presumably shipped in formaldehyde), projectiles, foreign bodies surgically removed and other items of interest for military medicine and surgery. Skulls were of particular interest because of speculation in the nineteenth century that the size of a person's skull determined intelligence. It's now a free museum open to the public called the National Museum of Health and Medicine, which has over twenty-five million bones, skulls, gory artifacts, preserved organs and assorted medical curiosities—including skull fragments and locks of hair removed during Abraham Lincoln's autopsy.

## *Further Reading*

Army Medical Museum, https://medicalmuseum.health.mil/.

Ifera, "Crime and Punishment, 1867–1891," 53–54.

Texas State Library & Archives Commission, "Moses Marshall."

Wooster, *History of Fort Davis*, 284–85.

## CHAPTER 16

# TEXAS WAS A GOOD PLACE FOR MEN, BUT AWFULLY ROUGH ON WOMEN AND OXEN

Women could not be soldiers in the frontier U.S. Army—but they were very much a part of army life. Officially, laundress was the only job a woman could hold for the army. Laundresses received a salary, fuel, a daily ration, living quarters, government transportation and medical care.

Even though very few personal accounts from army laundresses exist, since they were typically uneducated, census records show there were many, many laundresses. In fact, the army relied on them.

In 1855, one pregnant army laundress was traveling in Texas with the Eighth Infantry from Fort Duncan to Fort Chadbourne. She went into labor and gave birth in the back of a wagon. Meanwhile, the grass nearby had caught fire and was burning, but luckily, soldiers kept the flames from reaching her wagon—or the ammunition supply. Lieutenant Zenas Bliss described the event, using the polite term "sick" to mean "pregnant." He wrote, "We had no doctor along but some of the other laundresses attended the sick woman. There was a saying, ascribed to some female traveler, that 'Texas was a good place for men, but awfully rough on women and oxen.'"

Laundresses were part of the U.S. Army starting in 1802, adopted from the British Army model. Initially, one laundress did laundry for every twenty-five soldiers, and that was later changed to every nineteen and a half soldiers. Laundresses collected their pay directly at the pay tables before soldiers received their pay—the laundresses' portion having been deducted from each soldier's pay.

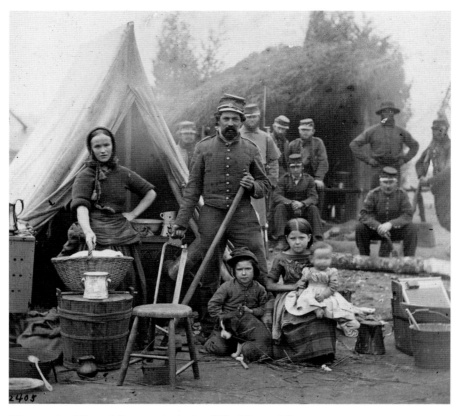

Women who followed the army had a hard life. *Library of Congress.*

In the 1870s, Congress began abolishing the institution of laundresses—trying to eliminate the burden of transporting women and their children along with wash tubs, scrub boards, wooden laundry paddles, heavy sad irons, pots and crocks for soapmaking, and assorted heavy washing equipment. In 1878 Congress decreed laundresses could no longer accompany troops, except at the discretion of the regimental commander; he might allow a laundress married to a soldier to remain with the troop until her husband's enlistment ended. In 1883 the army stopped providing rations to laundresses. Records in 1885 show that Fort Davis still had army laundresses.

Housing provided by the army for washerwomen was not prime real estate. At some forts, "Soap Suds Row" or "Laundry Row" or "Sudsville" denoted laundresses' quarters—usually located on the periphery of the garrison and often not far from a creek or river. This might be a collection

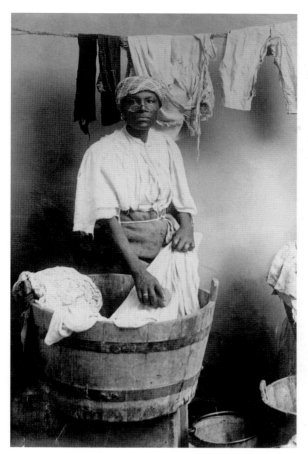

Laundresses played an important role at army garrisons. Being a laundress was tedious and hard physical work, but a laundress's monthly income could be more than a private's. Unfortunately, historical records provide no names for the people in either this photo or the one opposite. *Library of Congress.*

of huts, tents and sometimes barely habitable structures where laundresses lived. Women who did laundry at an army hospital were called matrons. It is not clear where hospital matrons lived—but records indicate that in the 1880s, the Fort Davis hospital complex included features such as a laundry, cistern, wood-house and matron's quarters.

So, who were these women? Barbara Millan was in her early twenties when she was a laundress/matron at the Fort Davis post hospital, from 1879 to the 1880s. Her sister Miguela (sometimes spelled Mecalia in old records) and her mother, Carmela (sometimes spelled Camila), were also hospital matrons there. Barbara married a European immigrant-turned-soldier named Anton Aggerman, who served with the Sixteenth U.S. Infantry at Fort Davis. Archives at nearby St. Joseph Catholic Church show Barbara and Anton were married by a priest in 1903. The church also has baptismal

**FACTOID** In the late 1800s, a laundress was paid 37½¢ per week per soldier. At that rate, if an industrious laundress washed for nineteen and a half men, she could earn $7.31 per week, or about $32 per month. That would make her monthly salary more than double that of an enlisted man, whose base pay was $13 per month. But the job of a laundress was physically taxing—plus, she had to make her own lye soap.

records of their children. According to the 1910 census of Jeff Davis County, Barbara was fifty-five and Anton was fifty.

During the Civil War, Susan Ann Baker—later known as Susie King Taylor—was officially listed on the army rolls as a "laundress." In actuality, she served as a nurse, cook and teacher for four years with the Thirty-Third U.S. Colored Troops Infantry Regiment, to which her first husband, Sergeant Edward King, was assigned. Serving with that Union regiment while in her teens, she also taught soldiers and others, including children, to read.

Born into slavery in Georgia in 1848, Susan was educated as a child at a clandestine school with the help of her beloved grandmother. When in her fifties, she published a noteworthy memoir about her experiences, "Reminiscences of My Life in Camp with the 33d United States Colored Troops, Late 1st S[outh] C[arolina] Volunteers." Writing of the horrors of battle, she says: "It seems strange how our aversion to seeing suffering is overcome in war, how we are able to see the most sickening sights, such as men with their limbs blown off and mangled by the deadly shells, without a shudder; and instead of turning away, how we hurry to assist in alleviating their pain."

In her memoir, she stated that she was never paid for her more than four years of service as an army nurse for the all-Black regiment. Nor did she receive a pension—same as the plight of other Black nurses in the Civil War. When the Civil War began, most nurses were men; women were considered too "frail" to cope with the challenges of handling the sick and injured. The profession of nursing was in its infancy, and there were no formal nursing schools in existence yet. In her book's closing, Susie King Taylor pleads eloquently for what came to be called civil rights, saying: "Justice we ask, to be citizens of these United States, where so many of our people have shed their blood with their white comrades, that the stars and stripes should never be polluted." She died at age sixty-four in 1912.

Another army laundress, Martha "Mattie" Howell Adams Collins, had six children by her first two husbands—having given birth to her first child at age fourteen. Then, in 1879, at Fort Concho, she married William J. Bishop, who worked for the army as a scout and civilian guide, and later he

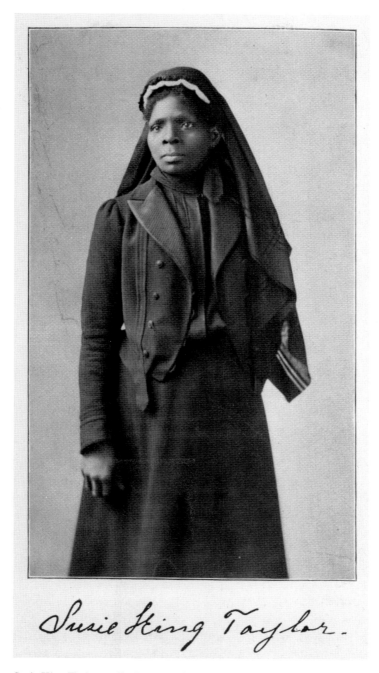

Susie King Taylor, earlier known as Susan Ann Baker. She was an army laundress, nurse, cook and teacher. Her memoir is remarkable. *Library of Congress.*

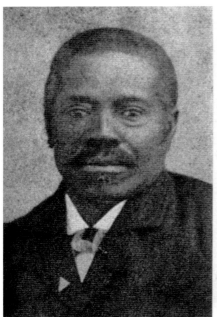 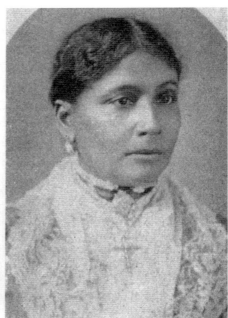

Sally and Menger Caldwell worked at Fort Davis for Major Anson Mills and family. *From* My Story *by Anson Mills.*

worked for the U.S. Army Quartermaster Department and as a civilian contractor for the army. In 1880, they moved to Fort Davis with the children; the youngest—their son, Bill—was born not long before that move. They had five more children, a total of twelve for Maggie.

At some point, they moved to a ranch south of Marfa on Alamito Creek. Even though she was not educated and signed her name with an *X*, Mattie raised sheep and goats and even some cattle for a while and had her own cattle brand. She is remembered as a hardworking pioneer woman of Irish descent, jolly, full of wit and a lover of nature, poetry and music; her husband played Irish tunes on the harmonica. Mattie Bishop lived out her life in Marfa and died in 1922. Her husband died the same year while working in Alaska.

Although not U.S. Army employees like laundresses were, some women also worked as domestic servants for army officers. Many servants, but not all, were women; some were soldiers called "strikers," and some were Chinese men. At times, officers' servants were Native American women, Black or White women, or European immigrants—or really, it was whoever was available. Officers' servants cooked, cleaned house, helped with childcare, washed and ironed clothes—typically for a salary of ten dollars per month, paid by the officer, which often included room and board.

Sally Caldwell was a domestic servant in the home of Major Anson Mills and his wife, Hannah. Both Sally and her husband, Menger Caldwell, a former soldier in the Tenth U.S. Cavalry, worked for the Mills family for eleven years, from 1882 to 1893, including at Fort Davis from 1882 to 1885. Mills wrote in his autobiography that he considered the Caldwells' service to his family "so capable and satisfactory" that he included their photos in his book. Unfortunately, he provided no other information about the Caldwells.

Most of the individuals who worked as laundresses, hospital matrons, nurses or domestic servants in officers' homes are unsung heroes. Their stories are yet to be told. Susie King Taylor is one of the exceptions, and her story is remarkable, yet she is typically left out of history books.

## *Further Reading*

Bishop (descendant/great-grandson of Mattie Howell Bishop; Fairfax City, VA). Communication with author.

Coffman, *Old Army*, 122.

Greene, *Historic Resource Study: Fort Davis.*

Jacobson and Nored, *Jeff Davis County, Texas*, 135.

Malburne, "Susie King Taylor, b. 1848."

Mills, *My Story*, 186, 200, 241.

Smith, Thompson, Wooster and Pingenot, *Reminiscences of Major General Zenas R. Bliss*, 53.

Stallard, *Glittering Misery: Dependents of the Indian Fighting Army*, 69.

Stewart, "Army Laundresses," 421–36.

Taylor, *Reminiscences of My Life in Camp*, 31–32, 75–76.

Thompson, *History of Marfa and Presidio County*, vol. 1, 157 and vol. 2, 239.

Wooster, *Frontier Crossroads*, 82–83.

## CHAPTER 17

# UNFIT FOR MILITARY SERVICE

## Why Do We Call It 4-F?

There were not many reasons to reject men being recruited to be soldiers in the Civil War. Both the Union and Confederacy needed all the men they could get.

There were, however, a few disqualifiers. The 1861 *Manual of Military Surgery* lists these conditions that rendered a man unfit for military service: hernia, epilepsy, paralysis, large tumors, bunions, bad corns, flat-footedness, hemorrhoids, anal fistula, spinal curvature, weakness of intellect, deformed fingers or hands, habits of intemperance, hydrocele/varicocele (swelling or enlargement in the scrotum or its veins) and defects of sight, hearing or speech.

Front teeth, also—they were very important for being a soldier. Starting in the Civil War, potential recruits were rejected if they did not have opposing upper and lower front teeth.

Why? At least four front teeth were needed to bite off the tip of the tough paper gunpowder cartridges used for muzzle-loading weapons. Molars in the back of the mouth would not work—only front incisors or canine teeth did the job.

Soldiers had to quickly bite and tear open the black powder cartridge with their front teeth, then put the powder and ball into the

**FACTOID** Before and during the Civil War, when preparing to fire a muzzle-loading rifle, a soldier ripped open the paper cartridge with his front teeth to expose the gunpowder. Next, he poured the powder into the rifle barrel, followed by the ball. Then he used the rifle's ramrod to force powder, ball and paper down the barrel.

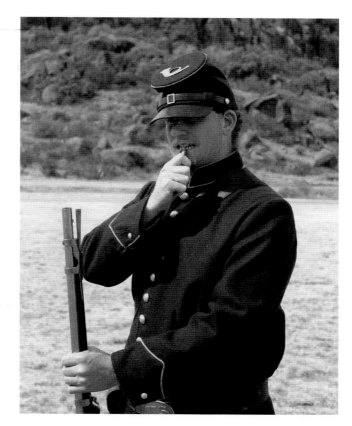

Civil War–era living history soldier at Fort Davis demonstrates tearing open a paper gunpowder cartridge. Having four front teeth was critical for a soldier to load his musket. *Photo by Max Kandler.*

barrel to fire the weapon. If a man could not perform this act of biting, he would not be able to load and reload his muzzle-loading musket in combat with comrades—thus putting them all at risk. At that time, routine dental care was nearly nonexistent, so sometimes even teenagers had teeth missing.

Thus evolved the term *4-F*—standing for "four front." Dental examiners of potential recruits rejected those who did not have four front teeth. When young men during the Civil War found out about this disqualifying factor, some had their front teeth pulled to avoid military service.

Since that time, 4-F has come to mean anyone not fit for service in the U.S. armed forces—for any reason whatsoever.

**FACTOID** Although toothbrushes were available by the late 1800s, brushing teeth was not common in America until after World War II, when soldiers—required to brush their teeth in the military—came home and continued the practice.

## *Further Reading*

Calcaterra, "4-F: Unfit for Service Because of Your Teeth."

Gross, *Manual of Military Surgery*, 1861.

Woodward, *Hospital Steward's Manual*, 1862.

## CHAPTER 18

# BRANDY, WHISKEY AND OPIUM TO TREAT TUBERCULOSIS

Pulmonary tuberculosis (TB) was the leading cause of adult death in nineteenth-century America. Many families lost loved ones to this dreaded disease, known as consumption. It struck rich and poor, young and old.

Most doctors at the time failed to recognize TB as a communicable disease, attributing it to factors such as heredity. After all, family members or people living in the same house tended to get the disease.

U.S. Army doctor Harvey Ellicott Brown had tuberculosis—also known as phthisis pulmonalis (pulmonary TB). Stationed at Fort Davis in 1881 as post surgeon, Brown was forty-five years old; his military tenure dated from before the Civil War. It is quite possible that he contracted the disease in the line of duty.

A rather interesting story unfolded—the way stories do. In August 1881, Dr. Brown's fellow officers at Fort Davis accused him of being "intoxicated" while serving on a court-martial board, and the army put him under arrest in his quarters. His rebuttal to the charge of intoxication was that he was merely treating his illness, which was causing him to cough violently and expel blood.

It is likely that Dr. Brown was treating his disease with beverage alcohol—i.e., whiskey or brandy—which would account for the charge of intoxication. Common treatment for TB at the time was one-half to one ounce of whiskey or brandy every two to three hours, or opium combined with beverage alcohol. Such a medicinal dose would render a person rather "relaxed"—but to a gentleman, the term "intoxicated" was an insult.

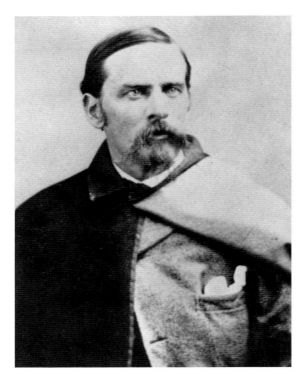

*Left*: Harvey Brown, MD, graduated from University Medical College of New York City. When he took the rigorous test to join the Army Medical Department, he filled out more than thirty pages writing answers longhand. *Fort Davis NHS.*

*Below*: Medicinal whiskey flask stamped "USA Hosp Dept." Army hospitals requisitioned whiskey, brandy and sherry wine for medicinal purposes. It could be dispensed in flasks such as this. *AMEDD Museum.*

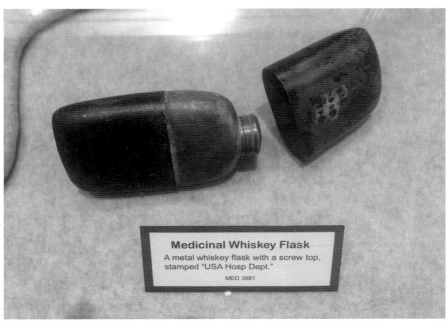

**Medicinal Whiskey Flask**
A metal whiskey flask with a screw top, stamped "USA Hosp Dept."
MED 3881

Two other army doctors at Fort Davis testified to Brown's sickness, saying that he suffered from "phthisis, second stage" and "gradual loss of flesh and muscular strength, frequent night sweats, persistent cough…general debility and depression of spirits."

With his trial looming large, Dr. Brown sent an urgent telegram to Assistant Surgeon General Charles Crane in Washington, D.C. He explained that he was not intoxicated but was very sick and that his health was rapidly declining. Crane telegrammed the Department of Texas medical director asking whether the charges could be dropped if Brown were removed from the department. The reply was yes.

So, the army dropped the charges and, after only five months at Fort Davis, transferred Dr. Brown to Jackson Barracks, Louisiana—a southern army post in a climate where he might not suffer so much from the ill effects of cold weather.

Five years later, in 1886, because of the debilitating effects of his disease, Dr. Brown requested to retire early. He was fifty years old. The adjutant general in Washington, D.C., denied Brown's petition, however, for the reason that even if he were found to be incapacitated, there was no vacancy on the army's retired list.

Still in effect was an 1861 law that limited "disability" to 7 percent of all regular army officers. Thus, it was difficult to obtain retirement for disability; a vacancy had to open up—i.e., someone on the list had to die—before an officer could be retired for medical disability.

So, Dr. Brown remained on the army's active duty rolls. He worked as a military historian, having already written a history of the U.S. Army Medical Department, published in 1873.

The ailing doctor died in 1889 in Louisiana, still on active duty and having the rank of major. He succumbed to TB—the disease he suffered from at Fort Davis eight years earlier, which was still untreatable by the best that nineteenth-century medicine had to offer. Buried at Chalmette National Cemetery, he was fifty-three.

## *Further Reading*

Fort Davis National Historic Site archival library, information on Harvey Brown, MD.

U.S. Army. *Registers of Sick and Wounded*.

## CHAPTER 19

# HOW TO LIMIT FAMILY SIZE:
# TWO WOMEN'S DILEMMAS

How might a nineteenth-century couple limit the size of their family? Primary sources reveal that Alice Kirk Grierson and her army officer husband, Benjamin, attempted to do so. Like many educated people at the time, they were prolific letter writers. In one letter, Alice mentions "an incomplete act of worship," probably referring to coitus interruptus (the withdrawal method): a common form of birth control in the nineteenth century.

The Griersons lived at various frontier army forts, including Fort Riley, Fort Concho and Fort Davis, but were at times separated due to his work in the field or to Alice being away on business or family visits. Living apart was certainly one effective method of birth control.

From Fort Sill, Indian Territory, in late 1871, Ben wrote Alice lovingly that he missed her and was lonely. She responded candidly that she wanted to stay longer in Chicago because she feared another pregnancy—as her last two births had brought on deep depression. Another time, in a letter to her faraway husband, Alice suggested in a genteel but very direct manner that it would be better if he did not come home because she did not want any more children.

It seems that whatever the Griersons did in order to limit the size of their family was not very effective, as Alice gave birth to seven children. (Or maybe it *was* effective—Alice herself was one of thirteen children.) Her childbearing stretched over seventeen years. She died in 1888 of bone cancer at age sixty.

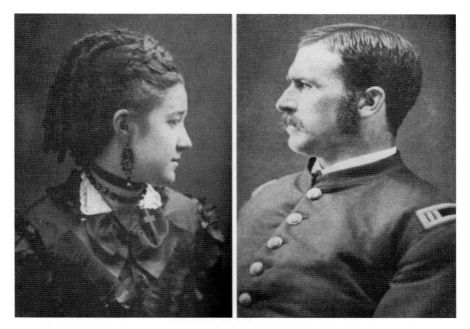

Emily McCorkle FitzGerald and Dr. Jenkins Augustus "John" FitzGerald. *Emily FitzGerald, An Army Doctor's Wife, University of Pittsburgh Press.*

At about the same time, 1874–75, another army officer's wife, Emily McCorkle FitzGerald, was writing letters home to her family in Pennsylvania from Sitka, Alaska. Emily's husband, army physician Dr. Jenkins Augustus "John" FitzGerald, was stationed there. They had two small children: two-year-old Bessie or Beth, born at West Point, and one-year-old Bertie, born in Sitka.

Emily's letters tell intriguing stories of life in Alaska, which the United States had purchased from Russia only seven years earlier in 1867. She was nervous about living in such a remote, mostly unsettled land and was concerned about her children's health, but she tried to remain optimistic. She described the Indigenous Tlingit people and the infrequent steamers—sometimes seven weeks apart—that brought food, passengers, supplies and mail.

Life was challenging, but the FitzGeralds were basically happy—except Emily worried about being so fertile. Apparently, pregnancy was a topic of discussion among officers' wives.

Emily was twenty-five in November 1875, when she wrote this letter from Sitka to her mother, Elizabeth:

*I have not been feeling well for a month. I know I look badly and I know Doctor* [her husband] *has been a little concerned, for he has put me on cod liver oil, and iron and quinine, and all those lovely things. I did not think I would tell you until I saw you, but I will now. I had a miscarriage about five or six weeks ago, but I lost a great deal of blood and all my strength. I nursed Bertie* [age one] *until about a week after it, and then I had to stop. I have not gotten over it yet. I guess the climate has a good deal to do with it, but I don't get strong as fast as I would like or Doctor hoped. I am thankful now that I did have it, as another Sitka baby would have been my fate. Now we know there won't be anything of that sort to fear, but Sallie* [Emily's sister] *need not trouble herself to have any. I can supply the family. I don't believe there is a safe day in the month for me. Indeed, I know there isn't.…Mrs. Campbell, Mrs. Field* [officers' wives], *and I have meetings of horror over the subject, as… we all seem to be awfully prolific.*

Next, the army transferred Dr. FitzGerald to Idaho, and the family lived at Fort Boise. Periodically, he served in the field on long, physically challenging assignments. Then, in October 1878, the FitzGerald family left Idaho and traveled to Pennsylvania. There, he reported to the Army Medical Board and was granted four months' leave.

After a happy time at Christmas spent with family, John became ill in January 1879 with "inflammation of the lungs" and was diagnosed with pneumonia. This was complicated by a wound he had sustained in the Civil War and a severe cold he contracted during the Nez Perce Campaign in Idaho.

**FACTOID** In today's age of instant electronic communication, writing letters as the sole method of communicating long-distance is hard for us to imagine. Yet that's what frontier people had—and thankfully so, because those letters give insight into a time long gone. What will future generations know of us who phone, text and email if we leave little or no record of our existence?

Dr. FitzGerald died seven months later at age forty, in August 1879, of "Consumption resulting from Pneumonia." Emily was twenty-nine. The following year, Emily filed for a widow's pension based on her husband's military service, but the army denied it on the grounds that (1) he had been on leave at the time of his death, and (2) his "fatal disease" was not contracted in the line of duty.

Emily hired a lawyer. Statements were gathered, such as a comment that her husband, the doctor, had made to his brother-in-law that "he had had

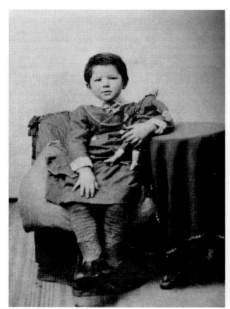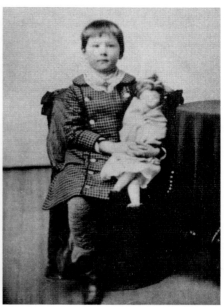

Herbert "Bertie" and Elizabeth "Bessie" FitzGerald in 1878. *Emily FitzGerald,* An Army Doctor's Wife, *University of Pittsburgh Press.*

a hard siege of service and took the worst cold of his life on the campaign and he feared one lung was seriously affected."

Emily's persistence paid off—eventually. Roughly ten years later, she began receiving a pension of $20 per month (about $400 nowadays). Pensions customarily included an additional small allowance for minor children, but by the time the pension board ruled in Emily's favor, her children were sixteen and seventeen years old. Emily died in 1912 at age sixty-one.

## Further Reading

FitzGerald, *Army Doctor's Wife on the Frontier,* 4–5, 165, 328–29.
Heitman, *Historical Register and Dictionary of the United States Army,* 1903.
Leckie, *The Colonel's Lady on the Western Frontier: The Correspondence of Alice Kirk Grierson,* 5, 61–62, 236.
Sitka History Museum, "Letters from Emily."

## CHAPTER 20

# WATER

## Where Will Our Next Drink Be?

**D**id you ever think what it was like traveling in a wagon train in the 1800s? These adventuresome trips were tediously slow, far from luxurious and certainly memorable—if you survived the months-long journey! Diaries of pioneers traveling in the mid-to-late 1800s in wagon trains going west—or east, because some returned—reveal sickness, death and trials of travel that we tend to forget about.

Harriet "Hattie" Bunyard was in her early twenties and single when she traveled from April to October 1869 with her family and others on the southern route from Collin County near Dallas, Texas, to Los Angeles, California. Her journal reveals intriguing details. It was a trip of about 1,400 miles—and it took them six months.

Hattie wrote that her wagon train consisted of eleven wagons, twenty men and eight families. There was no tally of the number of women. Near Fort Davis, she remarked about the high cost of corn at $1.50 per dozen ears, eggs at $1 per dozen and butter at $1 per pound. She described Fort Davis as "a pretty little place by the side of the mountains…a beautiful valley." She spoke of seeing "Negro" soldiers and hearing their band play as her wagon train passed the garrison.

Besides Fort Davis, they passed many army posts, abandoned or active—including Forts Richardson, Belknap, Phantom Hill, Chadbourne, Griffin, Concho, Quitman, Bliss, Cummins and Yuma. Hattie mentioned antelope, prairie dogs,

**FACTOID** In 1866, approximately one out of five soldiers in the U.S. Army contracted Asiatic cholera.

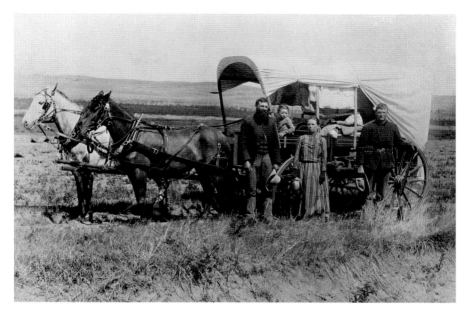

"Covered Wagon of the Great Migration." Travelers in wagons often stopped to resupply and repair equipment at army forts—the closest thing to our modern gas stations/ convenience stores. *National Archives; National Archives Identifier 518267; Federal Works Agency.*

native plants, Mexican travelers, a few "Indians," signs of "Indians" such as tracks and huts, as well as inconveniences like a broken wagon tongue. They traveled between nine and twenty miles per day. When the summer heat was oppressive for people and animals, the wagon train moved early in the day or at night.

When passing Fort Davis in June 1869, three months into the journey (which today would be a drive of about eight hours), Hattie's mother and fellow travelers suffered from "the Flux"—diarrhea or dysentery. Water was critical to the travelers, of course. Inadvertently, wagon trains promoted the spread of contagious diseases because such caravans of humans and stock animals like horses, mules, cattle and oxen repeatedly camped—and defecated—near the same water sources along the trails. Illnesses easily spread that were sometimes deadly, such as dysentery, typhoid fever and cholera.

**FACTOID** Quarantine as a concept came about in the Middle Ages as a practice of preventing ships from carrying plague to coastal towns. It's from the Italian words quaranta giorni, meaning "forty days."

**FACTOID** Advancing widespread acceptance of the germ theory of disease were John Snow (England), Joseph Lister (England), Louis Pasteur (France) and Robert Koch (Germany). The work of Ignaz Semmelweis (Hungary) in the 1840s proved fewer women died of puerperal or "childbed" fever after giving birth when obstetricians adopted a cleanliness protocol of handwashing and of disinfecting instruments—especially between doing autopsy work and examining patients. Semmelweis's observations and proposals were rejected by most in the medical community. Some physicians were offended by the suggestion to wash their hands, since they felt their social status as gentlemen guaranteed that their hands were clean. Others took pride in their bloodstained operating clothing, which was worn repeatedly. Semmelweis was ridiculed for proposing antiseptic procedures and was committed to an asylum in Vienna, where he died at age forty-seven in 1865—never knowing that his theories would help make drastic changes in medicine.

Since water was hugely important, Hattie often mentioned rain, springs, rivers, brackish water, water being sold by farmers along the road and, occasionally, a rain-filled pond or lake. Water could be treacherous, too. When crossing the flooding Pecos River, one of their mules drowned. Natural disasters impacting humans' lives are nothing new—but diaries like Hattie's are reminders of how vulnerable travelers in wagon trains were. Hattie, her parents and five siblings survived the journey. She died in 1897 in California at about age fifty.

Cholera was another disease that spread among travelers. In 1867, a cholera epidemic hit Fort Harker, Kansas—located on a busy westward trail—and it rapidly hit other forts and towns, leaving many people dead. At Fort Harker, U.S. Army doctor George M. Sternberg, age twenty-nine, buried his wife Louisa, age twenty, who died of cholera; when many civilians and army dependents were fleeing the area in fear, Louisa had stayed behind to help nurse the sick. One report says Louisa died six hours after contracting cholera. Another record states: "The surgeons were physically and psychologically distraught." Cholera often caused dehydration and fatal diarrhea, as well as violent vomiting and intestinal muscle contractions. Treatment included dosing patients with opiates and mercury compounds such as calomel, but not much worked. Now we understand that cholera is a bacterial infection—but when young Louisa Sternberg died of it in 1867, the science of bacteriology was just beginning in Europe.

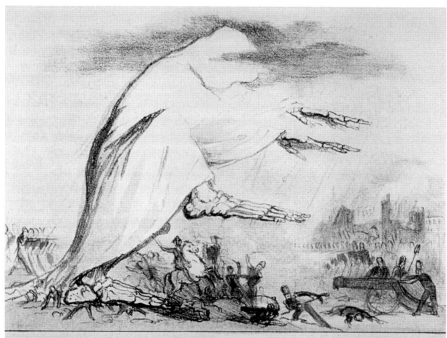

CHOLERA "TRAMPLES THE VICTOR & THE VANQUISH'D BOTH."

For centuries, people believed miasmas caused disease. This 1830s painting by Robert Seymour depicts poisonous air spreading disease during the cholera epidemic of 1832 that killed thousands of people in Europe and North America. *National Library of Medicine, NLM ID: 101393375.*

**FACTOID** In Italy in 1854, Filippo Pacini isolated the cholera bacterium while dissecting bodies during the Asiatic cholera pandemic (1846–63). But Pacini's work was not accepted by scientists and physicians because of the prevailing miasma theory, which held that disease was caused by "bad air" or poisonous vapors emanating from decaying organic matter.

Quarantine is how the Fort Harker garrison finally brought an end to the local cholera epidemic that travelers carried there, since most nineteenth-century doctors understood that diseases could be warded off by isolating and quarantining. Until late in the nineteenth century, however, few people had a clue that cholera is caused by water-borne bacteria entering the body through the mouth in drinking water or food.

When we complain about travel inconveniences today, we might remember nineteenth-century pioneers traveling without "luxuries" that we take for granted: paved roads, dependable clean water, heated or air-conditioned vehicles, cell phones for emergencies or convenience, hospitable hotels and restaurants along the way, electronic devices to entertain us and gas stations—with flush toilets, even!

## Further Reading

Carter and Carter, *Childbed Fever: A Scientific Biography of Ignaz Semmelweis.*

Craig, *In the Interest of Truth* […] *Life and Science of Sternberg*, 40–46.

Gillett, *Army Medical Department 1865–1917* and *Army Medical Department 1818–1865*, 11–12, 42.

Hastings, *Medicine: An International History*, 102.

Myres, *Ho for California! Women's Overland Diaries*, 196–252.

Pernick, *A Calculus of Suffering: Pain, Professionalism and Anesthesia in Nineteenth-Century America*, 11.

## CHAPTER 21

# YOU WERE BITTEN BY WHAT?

**A** raccoon bite was truly one of the most curious medical incidents at Fort Davis! This is one of those things the old Western films never portrayed.

It happened in February 1886 to a Third U.S. Cavalry trooper named Private Joshua Stallcup at a saloon just outside the military garrison of Fort Davis. The post surgeon wrote in the medical records that the soldier "was intoxicated when he was bitten by a pet raccoon."

So, here's the story. The saloon owner kept a pet raccoon, which no doubt helped attract customers, since raccoons are nocturnal—the same time when soldiers frequented bars. Also, since raccoons are noted for their cunning, intelligence and social behavior, their entertainment factor would be a plus for an enterprising business owner.

Whether the raccoon walked around the saloon or was kept in a cage is not known, but somehow, the raccoon bit the soldier—probably when he tried to touch it, pick it up, hold it or give it something to eat. Luckily, the animal did not have rabies or else the trooper would probably have died. The rabies vaccine had only been introduced to the world of medicine one year before, in 1885, by two French scientists, Émile Roux and Louis Pasteur.

No record exists to tell how post surgeon William H. Gardner treated the raccoon bite. Considering the state of the art of medicine at the time, he might have poured turpentine, ammonia or iodine on the bite and then released the soldier to regular duty. Or he might have splashed some medicinal whiskey on it—for that was in plentiful supply in the hospital storeroom—or given the soldier some to drink and sent him on his way. Tetanus shots were still unheard of.

Today, the soldier would have undergone a series of rabies shots if the raccoon were tested and found to have rabies. Private Stallcup's name does not appear in the Fort Davis death records, so he must have survived the raccoon bite.

# CHAPTER 22

# SURGERY AND ANESTHESIA

*urgeon* was a generic term used for centuries to denote a general practitioner. U.S. Army surgeons, in fact, performed few surgical procedures during the nineteenth century—except for during the Civil War. Other than that, army surgeons only performed surgery occasionally for minor things like anal fistula, foot surgery or finger amputation. In 1883, the annual report of the surgeon general in Washington, D.C., showed a total of 179 surgeries at all U.S. Army posts in the entire country—an average of one surgery per year per garrison.

Perhaps one factor in the low number of surgeries was that soldiers with serious conditions were simply discharged—sometimes at the rate of several per month at an army post. If a man could not perform the physically demanding duties, he was of no use to the army. Or maybe the low number of surgeries in the army reveals more about the state of medicine than anything else. Army doctors, like their civilian counterparts, were reluctant to operate for fear of infection. Antibiotics were years in the future. Without knowledge of what caused infection or disease, doctors were powerless in fighting it.

The use of anesthesia—ether, chloroform or nitrous oxide (ether)—began in the mid-1840s. Yet for years, some surgeons were reluctant to use it.

Anesthesia had drawbacks; ether was flammable, and chloroform sometimes caused cardiac arrest. Besides, it was very difficult to regulate dosage, and there was concern about adverse effects to the patient such as shock, poisoning, hemorrhage, pneumonia, lung irritation or circulatory failure.

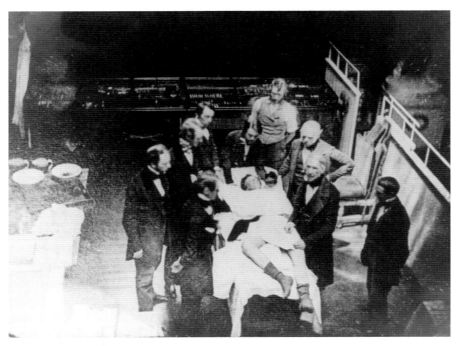

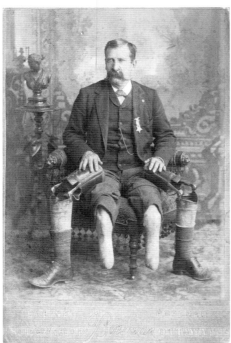

*Above*: Daguerreotype showing 1846 surgery using anesthesia in Boston. After a dentist administered ether, a surgeon performed neck surgery to remove a tumor. Favorably impressed, the physician afterwards said: "Gentlemen, this is no humbug." *Library of Congress.*

*Left*: Civil War veteran John W. January lost his legs to scurvy and gangrene while he was a prisoner of war at Andersonville Prison in Georgia. He is shown here in 1890 with prosthetic legs. *Library of Congress.*

**FACTOID** The expression "bite the bullet" may have originated from the military during a time when anesthesia was not available. Whatever its source, this idiom has taken on a broader definition and now simply means "to endure something."

A prevalent notion in the 1840s and '50s was that soldiers were—or should be—insensitive to pain. In the 1850s and 1860s, even after anesthesia was available, some surgeons continued to perform operations on non-anesthetized patients.

During the Civil War, military medical manuals for both the Union and the Confederacy recommended using anesthesia when available. Research shows it was used in the majority of Civil War surgeries—arm amputations being common—even though doctors at the time had limited surgical skills and often learned near the battlefield via on-the-job training.

Certain doctors were resistant to change. There were objections to the use of anesthesia in obstetrics on moral grounds. Some doctors believed that pain was beneficial and that anesthesia was biologically and emotionally unnecessary.

Physicians used anesthesia selectively, believing that individuals varied in their sensitivity to pain. A general theory was that children, women, the elderly, the affluent, and the educated were unable to endure pain, whereas males, Blacks, Native Americans, drunkards and people of lower economic classes had a high threshold of pain and could undergo surgery without anesthesia.

In the 1870s, anesthesia was popularly considered necessary only for major surgery. Minor surgical procedures that did not warrant anesthesia included cutting open the bladder to remove urinary stones, treatment for hydrocele (fluid in the scrotum), amputating fingers and toes, extracting small tumors, removing hemorrhoids and surgery on the jaw, throat, nose, eyes or anus.

By the 1880s, anesthesia was an accepted medical procedure, especially ether. Chloroform was losing favor because of its adverse effects on the heart. Things were changing as science revealed new information.

With increasing recognition in the late 1880s and early 1890s that disease prevention was related to cleanliness, some leaders in the medical profession began to urge surgeons

**FACTOID** In 1865, Joseph Lister (British surgeon/scientist) introduced the method during surgery of spraying carbolic acid on the surgical site to prevent infection caused by what we now know as microorganisms called germs. Thus was born antiseptic surgery. Then Louis Pasteur (French chemist/microbiologist) and Robert Koch (German bacteriologist) developed the germ theory of disease—which revolutionized the practice of medicine.

to prepare for surgery by methods such as the following: scrub hands in hot water for several minutes and soak them for three minutes each in hot solutions of potassium permanganate, then oxalic acid and finally bichloride of mercury. Rubber gloves were first introduced in 1889 as a measure to protect surgeons' hands from the caustic chemicals.

Medicine was advancing—slowly but surely.

## Further Reading

Bynum, *Science and the Practice of Medicine*, 121.

Gillett, *Army Medical Department, 1865–1917*, 49.

Lauderdale, "Letterbooks, 1885–1892, Vols. 8–9."

Pernick, *A Calculus of Suffering: Pain, Professionalism and Anesthesia in Nineteenth-Century America*, 35–39, 181–87.

Reimer, "Anesthesia in Civil War."

## CHAPTER 23

# CAMP FOLLOWERS CAME IN A WIDE VARIETY OF CHARACTERS

**L**ife on America's western frontier required an adventuresome spirit. Not everybody who went west did so because they chose to. Many men joined the army simply because it was a job. Others—like laundresses, entrepreneurs, military wives and "ladies of the evening"—followed the army. Life was rough, tough and dangerous, and some of the biggest enemies were disease and sickness.

Civilian jobs abounded when there was an army post nearby. Many different services were needed to provide logistical support on and off the post. The list in this chapter, taken from the 1880 U.S. Census, reveals the breadth of occupations.

**FACTOID** Gonorrhea and syphilis were treated with laudanum (opium) enemas, medications like mercury (calomel or blue mass pills), morphia, Dover's Powder (opium and ipecac), carbolic acid, iodides and guaiac (resin of a tropical tree), lotions to allay the pain and salt water baths or warm-water dressings to the genitals, as well as injections of lead, sulphate of zinc or nitrate of silver.

Old army medical records are proof that harlotry—prostitution—was alive and well near frontier army garrisons. There were plenty of cases of syphilis and gonorrhea among the troops that army surgeons treated. Throughout the 1880s at Fort Davis, army doctors treated over three hundred cases of venereal disease; they discharged soldiers with well-developed cases of VD.

Near the Fort Davis army garrison was a commercial enterprise built in 1883 by a businessman, James Watts. It had six to eight small rooms, which became known as "The Cribs"—probably a house of ill repute. Located in the area of town known as Chihuahua, it operated until the army closed the fort in 1891.

Also in 1883, two entrepreneurs named John Dunn and Fletcher Fairchild built a two-story saloon. Contents of the building included 360 bar glasses. This was a time when Fort Davis was at maximum strength, with about six hundred soldiers.

Dunn and Fairchild's saloon also had twelve spittoons, a large bar mirror, six beds with mattresses, six washstands with bowls and pitchers, seven mirrors, a billiard lamp and an ice refrigerator. We might call that an icebox—there was no electricity in town yet.

Listed among the saloon's contents was a gaming table known as Devil among the Tailors. This was a popular saloon game played with a ball attached to a pole and swung in an arc to strike the pins.

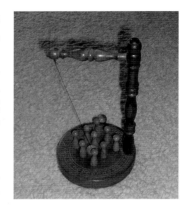

Devil Among the Tailors was a tabletop game played with a wooden ball (the "devil") suspended from a vertical post. The goal was to knock down the wooden pins ("tailors"). *Wikimedia Commons.*

Plenty of all types of women were around, despite the fact that women in general were a minority on the western frontier. Before the Civil War, an army doctor named Dr. Rodney Glisan felt strongly that the frontier was not a fit place for women. By the 1880s, however, things were changing rapidly in the American West. Women became opportunistic business entrepreneurs—including shopkeepers, laundresses, seamstresses and even "daughters of joy" (prostitutes) who inhabited or operated "hog ranches" (saloons/brothels) outside army posts.

The 1880 census records at Fort Davis list some women who operated businesses near or at the army garrison, such as:

A hairdresser, Alamia White, age twenty-eight, with rheumatism
A widowed shopkeeper named Dominga Learmas, age forty-one
A tailoress named Severona Mendoza
Manuella Urquedez, thirty-five, whose occupation was "keeps a dance house"
Eight seamstresses named Georgena Syareaz, Andria Yerzen, Leverana Salsodeo, Maria Gerzea, Rufia Valenzuela, Anetta Opez, Esta Gonzales and Fanny Harper

Women were a minority on the western frontier, and most soldiers were eager for the company of females. The U.S. Army discouraged marriage but allowed a small number of soldiers to marry—especially "long-service" men, often noncommissioned officers. Commissioned officers (lieutenants, captains and up) were allowed to be married. Officers' wives were regarded by the army as "civilizers" in the West—but they were not the ones who performed the crucial task of doing laundry for the military

In 1880, two-thirds of the population in the town of Fort Davis was of Mexican heritage, up from 50 percent in 1870. In the early 1880s, until 1885, most soldiers stationed at the garrison were Black. The 1880 census shows there were also people born in Belgium, Poland, Hungary, France, Switzerland, Germany, Scotland, Ireland, Wales, Denmark, Canada, the East Indies, the West Indies, Cuba, Australia and the Sandwich Islands (Hawaii). The census listed name, race, gender, age, occupation, schooling, whether people could read or write, place of birth, place of father's and mother's birth and physical infirmity—there was a column labeled "crippled."

**FACTOID** On the 1880 census, the oldest person listed—male or female—was age sixty; a few were as old as their early fifties. The overwhelming majority of residents were under age thirty, and there were lots of children. Many women were housekeepers, cooks or laundresses—some married to soldiers. Oddest of all was the census listing for Juanita Soutchez, thirty-five, whose line of work was listed as "idler." (One wonders if that's what she called herself, or if that's what the census enumerator chose to call her.)

Men's occupations in the 1880 census further reveal that Fort Davis was a diverse community. Some listed in town or at the fort were:

| | | |
|---|---|---|
| army druggist | cook | machinist |
| army officer | dance house keeper | merchant |
| army saddler | disabled soldiers (2) | messenger |
| army surgeon | farmer | milkman/dairyman |
| baker | gamblers (4) | musician |
| barber | gardener | plasterer |
| bartender | herder | post office clerk |
| blacksmith | hunter | restaurant keeper |
| butcher | judge | sailor |
| candy peddler | justice of the peace | school teacher |
| carpenter wounded by Indians | launderer | sheepman/shepherd |
| | lawyer | sheriff |

| | | |
|---|---|---|
| silversmith, born in Mexico | tailor | wagon boss |
| smuggler | teamster | wood chopper |
| station keeper | trader | |
| | U.S. soldier | |

Census takers surely met some fascinating people. What was a "sailor" doing in Fort Davis in 1880? One wonders what folks in the future will say about us when looking at twenty-first-century census records—it's doubtful anyone nowadays would tell a census enumerator that their occupation is "smuggler."

## Further Reading

Bartholow, *Practical Treatise on Materia Medica and Therapeutics* [1876], 169, 182, 232, 488.

Glisan, *Journal of Army Life*, 101.

Nored and Wiant, *Early Homes and Buildings of Fort Davis*, 19–20.

Stallard, *Glittering Misery: Dependents of the Indian Fighting Army*.

Wooster, *Frontier Crossroads: Fort Davis and the West*.

U.S. Census, 1880, Presidio County, TX.

## CHAPTER 24

# TRIALS OF A FRONTIER ARMY OFFICER'S WIFE

What an exciting young life Alice "Allie" Blackwood had. When she was only nine years old, in 1854, her family headed west to California from their home in Ann Arbor, Michigan. With her physician father, Thomas; her mother, Jane; her little sister, Mary; and an African American maid, Louisa, they traveled to Council Bluffs, Iowa. There they joined a wagon train of travelers and embarked on a six-month journey to California—mostly on the Oregon Trail.

Arriving in San Jose, California, her father began practicing medicine. Then they moved to Sacramento in hopes the climate might be more favorable for Allie's ailing mother. In 1856, after her mother died, Allie's father sent her and her sister back east, under escort of a clergyman and his wife, on a ship named the *Golden Age* that sailed from San Francisco to the Isthmus of Panama. Since this was almost six decades before the Panama Canal, the two girls crossed the isthmus overland on the backs of hired porters, who were referred to as "natives" in family letters.

Such adventures—all before Allie turned thirteen years old. At the Gulf of Mexico, they boarded another ship to New York City. From there, a train took them to Michigan to live with an aunt and uncle, where the two girls soon learned of their father's death. Teenage Allie began studying at the Young Ladies Seminary at Albion, Michigan—where she met two girls who were sisters to Frank Baldwin, Allie's future husband.

Allie, like many young single women looking for a husband, found the army officer's uniform appealing. In January 1867, she married twenty-

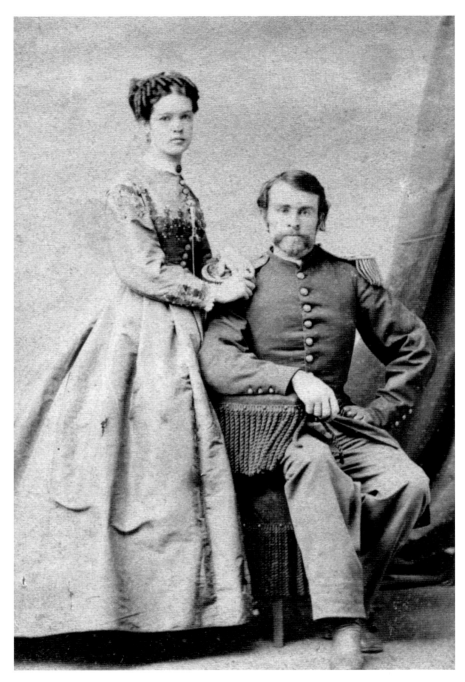

Baldwin wedding photo, 1867. Baldwin Collection, *Mossey Library, Hillsdale College.*

four-year-old Lieutenant Frank Baldwin and was eager to begin her life as an officer's wife. She soon learned, however, that it wasn't all excitement and thrills. "Glittering misery" is the term that some nineteenth-century officers' wives, like Martha Summerhayes and Kate Fougera, used to describe their lives.

Allie was twenty-two years old, bright, opinionated and trained to be a properly submissive Victorian lady in marriage. She dreamed of being a writer and a singer, but these dreams did not fit Frank's concept of an ideal army wife. Her husband expected her to dutifully and unquestioningly bow to the demands of his career.

Through the years, Allie suffered bouts of depression in her sometimes lonely, remote life on the western frontier, where she endured periods of separation due to the demands of Frank's duty. Frank himself struggled with alcoholism throughout his life. His two years as a POW in the Confederate-operated Libby Prison at Richmond, Virginia, during the Civil War likely impacted Frank's psyche, causing depression and anger and preventing a sense of inner peace—but at that time, society did not acknowledge the damaging psychological or physical effects of being a prisoner of war.

In September 1867, when Allie was seven months pregnant, the army transferred Frank from Fort Harker, Kansas, to Fort Wingate, New Mexico—and they began the thousand-mile journey overland with the army, traveling fifteen to twenty miles per day. On October 12, after a long and difficult labor during the lengthy wagon trip, Allie gave birth to Juanita, called Nita. This daughter would prove to be their only child. Even though Frank wanted a son, Allie's letters reveal she feared another pregnancy and the pain of childbirth.

Because there were no quarters available at the fort, Allie and the baby stayed at a boardinghouse in Lawrence, Kansas, while Frank went to Santa Fe in September 1869 to serve on a court-martial board. Allie wrote to Frank: "Frank, you can't imagine how lonely I am....Oh, for a home of my own with you and our baby."

The couple lived on Frank's army pay. In 1869, he received base pay of about $125 per month as a first lieutenant, or $1,500 per year.

In one letter to Frank when he was on field duty, Allie wrote that she had accepted an invitation to sing at a local Episcopal church, but Frank wrote back about his disapproval. Then, in her response to him, Allie told him that she had declined the offer yet expressed her extreme disappointment:

*Sometimes I feel bad to think, with the voice I possess, it can never have a higher sphere, a wider scope, than in singing always at home. It was a dear project of mine when I was a girl to make something of myself in vocal music, and I was so encouraged to do so and was succeeding so well in my efforts, and now it is all given up and all gone and my voice impaired with my disappointment.*

Two years later, on October 28, 1869, Allie wrote from Lawrence, Kansas, to Frank in Santa Fe:

*Mercy sakes what will I do if I have to stay here any longer without you and it is too bad little Nita is without her papa. I want her to know you and learn to love you. And Frank, I hope you love her as much as if she was a little boy. I know you…have always been greatly disappointed because she was not a boy, but she is an unusually smart and precocious child....She is as fat as butter, a perfect little dumpling.*

At Fort Leavenworth, Kansas, in September 1876, Allie asked her husband's permission to sing at a benefit that one of the officers' wives was having to help two German girls. Frank refused, lecturing Allie about what the proper role of an army wife was. He wrote:

*Be an ornament to…society, which you are fully competent and able to be, although you may not have all the finery that a few others may have, remember that true greatness lays in an honest, true, and upright heart, and feel, my darling, that you can by your interests in me and my welfare do a great deal to aid me....You know how much depends on a wife. I believe most fully she can and will cheer her husband in hours of darkness when his prospects are gloomy and improsperous.*

Allie wrote back to Frank: "I do try so hard to get along better than I do and to make the best of what I have and succeed so wretchedly and feel so discontented all the time."

In 1890, when Allie was forty-five, Frank wrote to her and asked if she would consider having another child. She responded in a letter dated November 26: "I think if I had a baby boy it would make us love each other more and I want one to please you and to please myself. I only dread the pain, darling, that's all. But if you can be with me I shall feel safer and happier....We will have a little boy Baldwin yet." At the time, Frank was stationed at Fort Davis, Texas, and was away on field duty—doing patrols and training missions in the canyons of the Big Bend.

A son was not meant to be, however, for Frank was called to South Dakota to assist with challenges due to resistance that Native peoples were giving the army. Allie remained behind at Fort Davis to arrange moving their possessions while the Army sent Frank to investigate the December 1890 Wounded Knee tragedy, in which several hundred Lakota were massacred.

Facing frustrations and challenges in his next work assignments, Frank struggled with health issues that likely stemmed partially from alcoholism and from his time as a prisoner of war during the Civil War. He served in the Philippines during the Spanish-American War, and when he reached the mandatory retirement age of sixty-two in 1906, he retired.

Letters reveal that Frank and Allie's marriage relationship was often disharmonious, exacerbated by Frank's alcoholism. Even when Frank and Allie reunited after being lonely while apart for military assignments, they often quarreled about social matters and Frank's professional advancement.

Their daughter, Nita, married an Englishman, Ambrose C.G. "Carlos" Williams-Foote, and they had four children—Baldwin, Gloster, Pierson and Alice. Initially, Frank disapproved of Nita's choice of a spouse. But then her husband joined the U.S. Army, earning Frank's approval. Nita also gave birth to a son, which Frank for years had longed for. In fact, Nita eventually had three sons. Finally, Frank acquiesced and came to accept the man his only daughter chose to marry.

Frank died at age eighty-one in 1923 in Denver. Cause of death was recorded as "cirrhosis of the liver." He had also suffered lifelong bouts of rheumatism. Allie died seven years later at age eighty-five in 1930 in Santa Monica, California, where Nita lived.

Having retired at the rank of major general after a long army career spanning the Civil War through World War I, Frank was the recipient of two Medals of Honor and had spent two years as a POW—yet, after he died, his wife of fifty-six years had to plead with the U.S. Board of Pensions to grant her a thirty-dollar monthly pension award.

In her final years, Allie wrote her memoirs, which she titled *Tales of the Old Army by an Old Army Girl* but which the publisher changed to

**FACTOID** "Some Rules by One Meticulous Army Officer for his Young Bride," 1869:

You will see that meals are served on time.

You will not come to the table in a wrapper [robe].

You will smile at breakfast.

You will not move the furniture without my permission.

You will do no work in the evenings. You will entertain me.

You will not touch my desk.

You will remember you are not in command of anything except the cook.

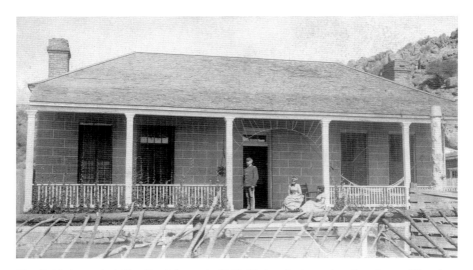

The Baldwins at their Fort Davis home in 1888. Today, the house is referred to as Historic Building 10 on Officers' Row. *Mossey Library, Hillsdale College.*

*The Memoirs of the Late Frank D. Baldwin, Major General, U.S.A.* The book was published in 1929, the year before she died.

Alice "Allie" Blackwood Baldwin and Frank Dwight Baldwin are buried side by side in Arlington Cemetery. It had been an eventful and challenging army career for Frank, including a yearlong work-related trip to Europe, during which time Allie met Queen Victoria—but one wonders how personally fulfilled Allie felt in the end.

## Further Reading

Baldwin (Alice Blackwood), *Memoirs.*
Carriker and Carriker, *Army Wife on the Frontier.*
Eales, *Living Within the Sound of Bugles.*
Fougera, *With Custer's Cavalry,* 15–22.
Reeder, "Some Rules," from *Born at Reveille.*
Steinbach, *Long March: The Lives of Frank and Alice Baldwin,* 1–3, 9–13, 48–49, 104–5, 149, 190.

## CHAPTER 25

# WHERE'S THE DENTIST?

A fourth-grade schoolboy from El Paso visiting Fort Davis National Historic Site in about 2003 noticed an old toothbrush on the ground near the ruins of an enlisted men's barracks. After being on the ground all those years, the toothbrush was just a weather-worn, wooden handle! The bristles were gone, but holes remained where bundles of natural bristles had been—probably made of boar's hair or horsehair.

It had been over one hundred years since the U.S. Army departed Fort Davis in 1891. The toothbrush was lying close to one of the barracks, where a soldier might have dropped it.

Who knows how many soldiers had a toothbrush. The army did not issue toothbrushes, but they were available at shops for as little as 6¢—however, for a soldier whose salary was $13 a month, that's not as cheap as it seems! (The value of 6¢ in 1885 would be about $1.60 today.)

In America, a toothbrush was first patented in 1857, and by the mid-1880s, toothbrushes were being mass produced. Bristles of early toothbrushes were made of pig or hog hair or even horsehair, set in a handle made of wood, bone or celluloid.

There's an entertaining toothache story that took place in 1877 at Fort Abraham Lincoln, Northern Dakota Territory. A soldier walked into the post hospital dispensary holding his lower jaw, moaning and complaining of an aching tooth. He asked for some chloroform to numb the pain so the hospital steward could pull the tooth.

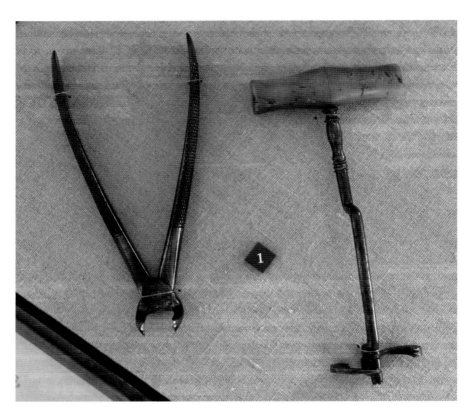

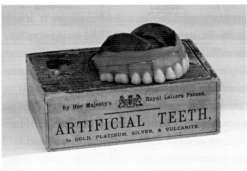

*Above*: Private Mulford probably had his tooth pulled in 1877 with one of these dental instruments of the period. *Fort Davis NHS.*

*Left*: Early dentures made of vulcanite were affordable to common folk. *British Dental Museum, London.*

Meanwhile, out the window, he watched an officer's wife and an army laundress walk past one other, each driven by intense curiosity to turn back and gawk at the other's dress. The laundress resisted the urge to do so, but the officer's lady turned to look and, in so doing, tripped over a wheelbarrow and fell down, losing her hat—and her pride. She ended up on the ground in an unladylike position, exposing her striped stockings, with the wheelbarrow in her lap. Quickly regaining her composure, she stood up and indignantly kicked the wheelbarrow, then continued on her way.

The soldier with the toothache laughed heartily. He was so amused that his toothache disappeared, and he tolerated the hospital steward pulling the tooth without chloroform, which he called "the go-to-sleep." According to Private Ami Frank Mulford, who told the tale in his memoirs, the hurting trooper remarked: "Steward, never mind the go-to-sleep. Haw, haw, haw. Get your forcips [*sic*] and yank that tooth right out quick. Hee-he, haw-haw! I'm tickled to death and the tooth is asleep. He-haw! Out with her before she wakes up!"

One more toothache story gives insight into life before the routine dental care that we take for granted. Even as a young army bride at the age of twenty-two in 1867, Alice "Allie" Blackwood Baldwin, wife of Lieutenant Frank Baldwin, suffered decaying teeth. She tried to keep her mouth closed much of the time because her teeth had decayed badly.

In a letter in October 1869 to her husband when he was away, Allie mentioned she hated the way her rotten teeth ruined her smile and fouled her breath. Suffering great pain, she found a dentist to pull all her teeth and fit her with dentures. She wrote: "Ain't you glad they are out, Frank, so now you won't smell my awful breath any more?" At the time, dentures were typically porcelain teeth set in a frame made of flexible-then-hardened rubber, known as vulcanite—a compound that Charles Goodyear discovered how to make in the 1840s. Finally, artificial teeth were no longer a luxury just for the rich.

## Further Reading

Mulford, *Fighting Indians! In the Seventh U.S. Cavalry*, 51–52.
Steinbach, *Long March: The Lives of Frank and Alice Baldwin*, 26, 49.

## CHAPTER 26

# YOUR TB TREATMENT IS SCHEDULED FOR TWO O'CLOCK IN THE INHALATORIUM

I t's unfortunate that army surgeon Dr. Harvey Brown (chapter 18) died at a time of transition in medical understanding of the disease that killed him, tuberculosis. In 1882 in Germany, microbiologist and physician Robert Koch discovered that infectious bacteria caused TB—and that it was a communicable disease, not one linked to genetics.

Since there was not yet a real cure, many doctors recommended that people with such respiratory conditions go to sunny, dry, cool climates at high elevation in the American West.

One such place was Fort Davis. Starting in the late 1880s and continuing through the early 1900s, people with respiratory conditions came to Fort Davis for its high desert climate, which was considered to be healthy for people suffering from breathing ailments.

At some point after the army deactivated the Fort Davis garrison in 1891, two men named Will Pruett and E.H. Carlton established a

**FACTOID** Tuberculosis was the main cause of death in America in the late nineteenth century and at the turn of the twentieth century. Many doctors believed it was a hereditary condition. One popular treatment was to send TB patients, called "lungers," to live in tents in high, dry climates with lots of fresh air and sunshine, like Fort Davis or certain areas of New Mexico. Scientists began to realize in 1882 that TB was caused by communicable infectious bacteria. Some of the first sanatoriums were created by the federal government at abandoned military forts, like Forts Bayard, Lyon and Stanton, to isolate and treat sick soldiers and veterans.

tubercular sanitarium known as Tent City. Some say this was around 1908. Located a few miles east of town, the sanitarium reportedly had twelve cottages and a dining/recreation hall.

An interesting medical feature of Tent City was the "Inhalatorium," a large metal box like a booth with windows. Inside, a sick patient sat and breathed a liquid mixture containing camphor, carbolic acid and salt gum. This same principle was later adapted as a nebulizer.

Tent City was in operation for only a few years. As understanding about pulmonary TB grew, people found medical treatments in urban locations, and Tent City became defunct.

Of course, the Inhalatorium treatment was only palliative—it did not cure tuberculosis. Even with powerful antibiotics today, there's still not a magic cure for TB. Resistant strains continue to evolve for this disease that has been around since antiquity.

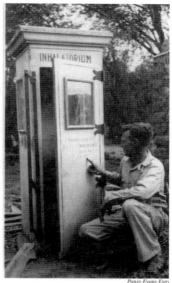

*Pansy Evans Espy*

Dick Swartz examines "Inhaletorium" from "Tent City".

Tent City inhalatorium. TB patients sat in a zinc-lined chamber for breathing treatments; drugs were administered via steam vapor. *Fort Davis NHS and Jeff Davis County, Texas.*

## Further Reading

Jacobson and Nored, *Jeff Davis County, Texas*, 157–59.

## CHAPTER 27

# DEATH HOVERED CLOSE FOR WOMEN IN CHILDBIRTH AND FOR CHILDREN

In 1880 at Fort Concho, when an officer's wife gave birth to a dead child, Alice Kirk Grierson, the post commander's wife, said she heard rumors—that women wearing corsets could be the cause of babies being born dead. Corsets, at the time, were standard wear for Victorian ladies, even in pregnancy.

Another tragic twist of fate, like the death of newborns, was a fairly common event—when a mother died giving birth. One woman who died in childbirth was Margaret Ann "Mary" Gear Carpenter, first wife of Captain Stephen Decatur Carpenter. She died in 1852 at Fort Terrett, Texas, and was only twenty-nine or thirty years old. She and the newborn, Gilbert, were buried there. Then, after Fort Terrett closed, the bodies were moved to Fort McKavett. At the time, Mary and Stephen had a four-year-old daughter, Alice.

Stephen remarried four years later. His new wife was Laura Clark of Maine, who at age twenty-five had traveled by ship, the *T.M. Fannin*, from New York to Galveston, Texas, to be a schoolteacher. It was a trip of 1,800 miles by water and took thirty days. From Galveston, Laura took a steamer to Brazoria on the Brazos River and taught on a plantation that grew sugar and cotton, using slave labor to do so. Her salary was $250 a year, including "board" (meals). Laura's letters home reveal that she was suffering from a respiratory condition.

When she met West Point graduate Stephen Carpenter, he was an army officer at Camp (later Fort) Lancaster, Texas. They traveled to Maine to get married, then returned to his duty station at Fort Lancaster. In 1858, Laura wrote letters to Stephen, who was away on detached service, and mentioned ten-year-old Alice, who was with Laura and whom Laura loved as her own. After Stephen's military leave, when they traveled to Maine for a holiday, during the fall of 1859, Stephen and Laura returned—this time to Fort Stockton, Texas—but they left Alice with family back east. Laura's poor health likely played into that decision.

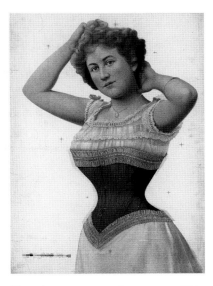

Victorian woman wearing a corset. This is the body shape that women of the time period aspired to. *Library of Congress.*

Then, in November 1860, Laura died—not long after giving birth to a son, John, at Fort Stockton, Texas. She was thirty-four. Her death was due to complications of childbirth, compounded by serious lung problems and tuberculosis. Stephen hired a nurse for the child, then took him to Maine, where the next year, the nine-month-old infant died.

Two years later, Major Stephen Carpenter was killed in action during the Civil War at the Second Battle of Murfreesboro, Tennessee. At five feet, eleven inches tall, he must have been a striking figure on horseback—when six Confederate bullets slammed into him and ended his life at age forty-four. Little Alice Carpenter lived with a Gear family relative of her birth mother. She married, had two children and died at the age of twenty-nine.

Before 1900, about one in three babies died. If children could just make it to adulthood, avoiding illnesses and childhood diseases like measles and diphtheria, they had a pretty good chance of surviving. Sad stories abound with tales of infants dying.

In 1857, Captain Arthur Tracy Lee and his wife, Margaret, buried their fifteen-month-old son at Fort Lancaster. At the time, Lee, who was stationed at Fort Davis with the Eighth U.S. Infantry, was returning with his family from military leave in San Antonio when the baby took sick along the way. The little one died at Fort Lancaster.

A somber funeral was held, and people at the small army garrison offered consolation to the grieving parents. In his July 1857 diary entry about the child's death, young Lieutenant May Humphreys Stacey, who had stopped with the U.S. Army Camel Corps at Fort Lancaster, wrote:

> *We were all very sorry, and sympathized deeply with the captain and his poor wife. For her our sympathy was particularly lively. There she was in the wilderness, or at a frontier post, with only two or three of her own sex, and they entire strangers. They could not feel or appreciate a mother's grief, like one who had an acquaintance with Mrs. Lee before.*

## Further Reading

Dixon, "Letters from Texas: An Army Wife on the Texas Frontier," 181–97.
Green, *The Dancing Was Lively: Fort Concho, Texas*, 90.
Stacey, Beale and Lesley, *Uncle Sam's Camels* [...] *1857–1858.*

CHAPTER 28

# SUDDEN DEATHS

I n 1856, an infantry soldier named John Freeland at pre–Civil War Fort Davis suddenly dropped dead, no doubt leaving his fellow soldiers stunned. After an autopsy, post surgeon Andrew Jackson Foard logged this in the medical records: "Perfectly healthy up to the time of his death. After dinner, he sat smoking his pipe by the fire in the company barracks; got up to go outside and fell on his face, dead. Post mortem showed ¾-inch rupture of right auricle; pericardeum distended. The man was a heavy drinker."

On the death record, the doctor gave the cause of death as "rupture of the heart." Like most soldiers at the time, Private Freeland was a young man.

So, might the army doctor have diagnosed or foreseen this and helped the soldier take steps for prevention? Well, who knows? Diagnostic tools in the 1850s consisted of a physician's training, experience and intuition—as well as books and often a skeleton hanging in the surgeon's office or other room at the post hospital. Diagnostic tools such as X-rays, MRIs and CT scans were in the future.

A skeleton was a great reference tool, to be sure—yet it's kind of creepy for us to think of seeing an actual human skeleton hanging there, since we are accustomed to mere charts hanging in doctors' offices. One wonders where or how the nineteenth-century army procured human skeletons for its military hospitals.

A bizarre event for Fort Davis was the day lightning struck and killed a cowboy named John Drinkwater—as well as his horse—when he was

*Right*: Life-size plastic skeleton in restored post surgeon's office at Fort Davis. In the 1800s, it would have been actual human bones. *Photo by author.*

*Middle*: Lightning blew a hole in the hat of twenty-year-old British cowboy. It struck and killed him as well as his horse near Fort Davis, 1885. *National Museum of Health and Medicine.*

*Bottom*: The 1888 Hospital Corps classroom at Fort Union, New Mexico, had a skeleton for training purposes. After the army established the Hospital Corps in 1886 to provide better training to hospital personnel, most post hospitals likely had a classroom similar to this. *Fort Union National Monument, New Mexico.*

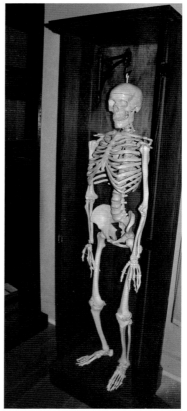

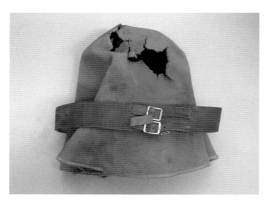

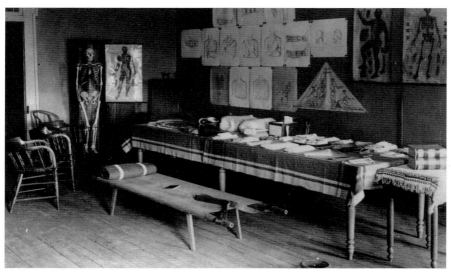

riding in a thunderstorm in August 1885. He was twenty years old, probably hurrying to get out of the rain.

Since Drinkwater was a civilian who died outside military garrison boundaries, civil authorities summoned the only doctor in the area, army post surgeon William H. Gardner, to examine the body. In payment for his services, they gave him Drinkwater's hat—showing a hole where the lightning struck. Dr. Gardner had lost a colleague to a lightning strike when they were in medical school together before the Civil War, so perhaps he had a personal interest in lightning. He soon shipped off the hat to the Army Medical Museum in Washington, D.C.

According to local folklore, they buried John Drinkwater on the hill east of town where lightning tragically ended his young life. This was reportedly near the spot where Hillcrest Cemetery is today.

## Further Reading

Jacobson and Nored, *Jeff Davis County, Texas*, 197.
Lauderdale, "Letterbooks, 1885–1892, Vols. 8–9."

## CHAPTER 29

# MEDICAL WHISKEY AND OTHER ELIXIRS, NOSTRUMS AND CURE-ALLS

T he post hospital had a ready supply of liquor. Many diseases were treated with brandy or whiskey or wine. Nineteenth-century doctors treated symptoms to give the patient comfort—that was the state of the art of medicine. The Fort Davis Medical Inspection Report of April 1886 revealed that liquor was "prescribed freely for patients with drinking habits, [or] down in bed with pneumonia, typhoid fever, etc."

Two popular misconceptions about alcohol contributed to its use: (1) When ingested, alcohol will kill disease and (2) Alcohol has food value, since it's often made from grain, fruit or vegetables. Both wrong—but thus evolved the terms *beverage alcohol* and *medicinal alcohol*.

Army hospital stores included medicinal alcohol in the form of big, thirty-two-ounce bottles of whiskey, sherry wine and brandy. At Fort Davis, these were kept locked— along with powerful morphia, alkaloids and strychnia—in the hospital storeroom building near the hospital. Guess who guarded the key: the hospital steward.

In 1871, post surgeon Daniel Weisel complained about his drunk hospital stewards

**FACTOID** One nineteenth-century medical doctor wrote that alcohol/liquor was generally accepted as "a stimulant to digestion, a cardiac tonic, a conservator of tissue, capable of increasing and sustaining the vital energy, and…indispensable in the treatment of all lower grades of disease, shock, collapse, etc." Brandy was used historically to ward off plague and in the nineteenth century was a medicine for blood pressure and the heart.

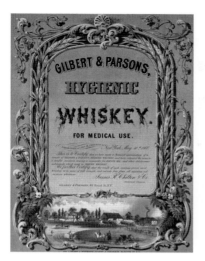

"Hygienic Whiskey for Medical Use," 1860. Doctors prescribed whiskey frequently to treat medical conditions, but the army hospital's medical supply was kept under lock and key to prevent overindulgence. *Library of Congress.*

having easy access to the army medical supply of brandy and whiskey. He charged the two hospital stewards, Fred W. Wearick and Lucius G. Currier, with disobeying orders and neglecting their duties— misappropriating medicinal alcohol and possibly pilfering money from the hospital fund. The army held a trial for both men and dishonorably discharged Currier.

Wearick continued working as a hospital steward at Fort Davis, and apparently, he kept up his pattern of "misappropriating" hospital liquor intended for medical purposes. In 1877, he was found guilty of stealing 125 bottles of whiskey, brandy, wine and other alcohol from the hospital storeroom.

One rather amusing incident happened when an inebriated officer named Lieutenant John M. Cunningham went to the Fort Davis post hospital on November 19, 1889. He boisterously demanded that the hospital attendants give him "aromatic spirits of ammonia." Arriving at the hospital in a half-clad condition without shoes or coat, talking incoherently and acting violently, Cunningham was locked up in the fifteen-foot-square isolation room "to get sober." When the frenzied lieutenant broke windows and flourished a knife, the officer of the day put Cunningham in a cell at the guardhouse overnight. The next day, he was returned to the hospital isolation room with a sentry posted at the door. At one point he escaped, grabbed an iron bar and went after the sergeant who put him in the guardhouse. Surely, there were many such stories at military posts about inebriation due to the "medicinal alcohol" or "beverage alcohol" used to treat a variety of medical conditions, as well as those with drinking problems. Besides, it was no doubt common knowledge that the post hospital had supplies of whiskey, wine and brandy for medical purposes—including the treatment of asthma.

At the frontier post of Vancouver Barracks, Washington, in 1894, army surgeon Dr. William H. Arthur found an effective way to cure drunken behavior. He treated the intoxicated soldier as if he were suffering from poisoning. Inserting a perforated wooden gag in the drunk soldier's mouth,

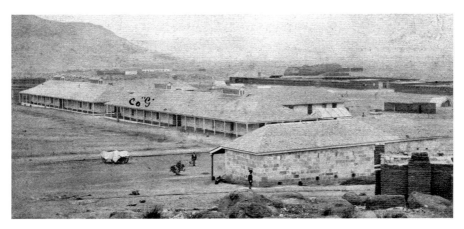

Fort Davis in 1871, with enlisted men's barracks and stone guardhouse (*foreground*). This guardhouse was replaced in 1882 due to overcrowding, poor ventilation and escapes. *Courtesy John Patterson Lindley.*

and with the help of two or three hospital attendants to hold him down, the doctor thoroughly pumped the man's stomach. Though painful, Dr. Arthur felt this was sometimes an effective way to curb drunken behavior.

## *Further Reading*

Clary, "Role of the Army Surgeon in the West: Daniel Weisel."
Coffman, *Old Army*, 388.
Ifera, "Crime and Punishment, 1867–1891," 167–69.
Jacobson and Nored, *Jeff Davis County, Texas*, 69.
Rothstein, *American Physicians in the 19th Century*, 194–95.

## CHAPTER 30

# TAKE A PHOTO OF OUR BELOVED DAUGHTER–SHE'S DEAD

**D**isease and sickness were great equalizers. No one was immune, not even a high-ranking army officer's daughter.

Typhoid fever took the life of young Edith Clare "Edie" Grierson at Fort Concho, Texas, on September 9, 1878, not long after her thirteenth birthday. Probably no one connected the cause of her death to the drinking water, which the garrison drew from the Concho River and from a spring—both of which were contaminated by animal fecal matter.

The army doctor treated young Edie's swollen tonsils by "touching them with caustic" (probably a toxic medicinal substance such as creosote or carbolic acid) and giving her injections of quinine for fever. Edie was vomiting, and the week before her death, she took no solid food and was living on "wines, brandy, & essence of beef injected into her bowels."

Even though the death of a child was not uncommon at frontier army posts, the Fort Concho post commander, Colonel Benjamin Grierson, and his wife, Alice, were devastated to lose their only daughter. They had done everything to save her, including sending a telegram to Fort Worth for ice, which took five days to arrive—a distance of over two hundred miles. Chewing ice gave the dying girl comfort.

After Edie's death, her parents did what many people did at the time, especially for dead children: they hired a traveling photographer to take pictures of the deceased person before burial. In this case, the photographer was M.C. Ragsdale, and his postmortem photos served as keepsakes for the Grierson family and friends.

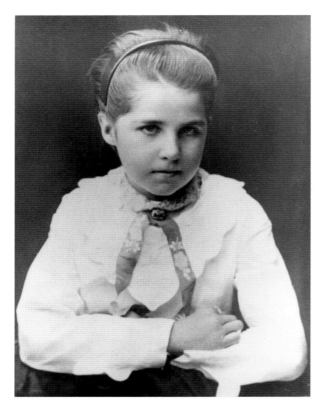

*Left*: Young Edith Grierson before her untimely death. *Fort Concho NHL photo archives.*

*Below*: Postmortem photo of Edith Grierson, who died of typhoid fever at Fort Concho in 1878. *Fort Davis NHS.*

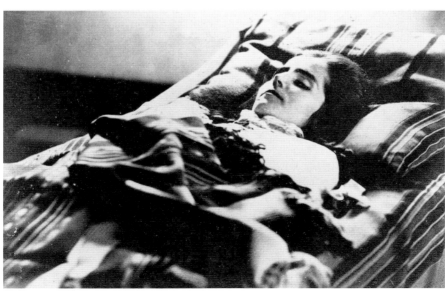

It is rather gruesome for us today to see the photo of a dead person lying serenely as if sleeping. Postmortem photography was popular then. This was before personal cameras became accessible.

After Edie's burial in the Fort Concho Post Cemetery, her mother, Alice, mailed letters to close relatives and friends telling of Edie's death, and she included postmortem photos—including the one shown here.

Many people worldwide died of typhoid fever before there was an understanding about waterborne illness. The year after young Edie Grierson's death, the army post of Fort Concho in San Angelo installed an improved water system.

**FACTOID** Some say Edie's ghost still visits the Grierson home on Officers' Row at Fort Concho where she died. She has been seen playing her favorite game, jacks. When there's an apparition, the room feels chilly, and Edie turns her head to smile at visitors. Items in the room are sometimes moved around, and people hear footsteps walking on the stairs, a door slamming, a ball bouncing or other strange sounds. Why not? Her life was cut short prematurely.

## *Further Reading*

Leckie, *The Colonel's Lady on the Western Frontier: The Correspondence of Alice Kirk Grierson*, 115–19.

## CHAPTER 31

# DEMON WHISKEY

**A**lcoholism was a serious problem in the nineteenth-century U.S. Army. Until 1830, whiskey was actually part of the ration. After that, the army sometimes issued whiskey to extra-duty soldiers and on occasions like Christmas.

To escape the monotony of life at isolated frontier garrisons, enlisted men and officers alike turned to whiskey and beer. At one point in the 1880s, there were reportedly as many as thirteen saloons in town near the army post of Fort Davis.

Alcohol is "the curse of the army," wrote Private James B. Wilkinson, Second U.S. Cavalry at Fort Assiniboine, Montana Territory, in the mid-eighties. The *Annual Report of the Secretary of War* in 1891 indicated that throughout the 1880s, nearly one out of every twenty-four men were hospitalized as alcoholics. To have been put in an army hospital means it was serious.

Certainly, a ready supply of alcohol contributed to drunken behavior. For years before the Civil War, the sutler's store—and after the Civil War, the post trader's store—monopolized business at army garrisons. They typically sold liquor by the drink or by the bottle. Forts often had both an officers' bar and a soldiers' bar on the premises, as well as sometimes a billiard table or two.

In 1881, however, U.S. president Rutherford B. Hayes—pressured by teetotalers—abolished the sale of hard liquor on military garrisons. Soldiers started going off-post to what were sometimes less than respectable private

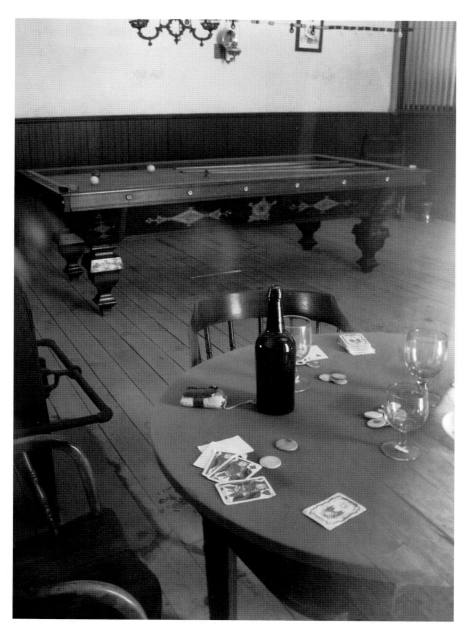

At Fort Laramie, Wyoming, restored officers' bar room on post. *Photo by author.*

saloons, often known as "hog ranches." There, proprietors sold inferior-quality whiskey, encouraged gambling and sometimes provided prostitutes. Then, in the mid-1880s, attempting to control drunkenness and unhealthy or immoral behavior, the U.S. Army established canteens on-post, where soldiers could purchase and consume drinks in a controlled manner on the garrison grounds.

At the canteen, the government subsidized food, drinks and recreation. Canteens were more affordable for soldiers than the price-gouging, off-post establishments. Originally a British army concept, the canteen was a combination snack bar and rec hall where soldiers could buy a beer, recreate, get something to eat and just relax.

By the mid-to-late 1880s, Fort Davis had a post canteen, located in what was once the mess hall wing of an unoccupied barracks (now referred to as Historic Building 23). An army inspection report at Fort Davis in March 1890 stated that the canteen boasted a gymnasium. It is unknown what gym equipment it contained or what funds purchased the equipment. Perhaps profits from the canteen went toward the purchase.

Twenty years earlier, in 1869, Fort Davis post surgeon Dr. Daniel Weisel had advocated physical exercise for the troops. Reporting that there was no gymnasium, he argued that a gym would improve the physical and moral condition of the soldier by providing "innocent and healthful amusements and lessening his inducement to side pleasures farther away and more injurious." It took twenty years for Dr. Weisel's dream to come true, and it happened just a year or two before the army closed Fort Davis.

The canteen at Fort Davis had two large rooms—one with a lunch counter and three billiard tables, and the other for playing games like backgammon, chess and cards. As with the benefits that baseball provided, the army soon found that when there was a canteen on-post, morale and discipline improved. Plus, an inspection report in summer 1890 revealed: "A swimming pool is now in course of construction" (probably an area in Hospital Canyon where the rainwater drainage collected behind large boulders).

Canteens at remote frontier army posts definitely made life more bearable. In later years, the canteen evolved into the post exchange or "PX"—first established in 1895 by presidential order. This put an end to the era when sutlers and post traders sometimes took advantage of being the only shops available to soldiers and charged exorbitant prices.

One frontier army officer's wife, Martha "Mattie" Dunham Summerhayes, summed up the positive benefits of an army canteen:

*The men were contented with a glass of beer or light wine, the canteen was well managed, so that profits went back into the company messes in the shape of luxuries heretofore unknown; billiards and reading rooms were established....The men gained in self respect; the canteen provided them with a place where they could go and take a bite of lunch, read, chat, smoke, or play games with their own chosen friends, and escape the lonesomeness of the barracks.*

## Further Reading

Coffman, *Old Army*, 359–60.
Greene, *Historic Resource Study: Fort Davis*, 150.
Rickey, *Forty Miles a Day on Beans and Hay*, 156, 159, 168.
Summerhayes, *Vanished Arizona*, 259.
Weigley, *History of the United States Army*, 270.

## CHAPTER 32

# CHILDREN DIED, TOO—AND THERE WERE NO CHILD-PROOF CAPS

**B**abies and children died at frontier army posts, but their deaths do not generally show up in official military or medical records.

At Fort Davis, it wasn't until the 1880s that the post chaplain began to record civilian deaths. On June 30, 1886, reports indicate that a soldier's child "died from poison" or as a result of "opium poisoning." Fifteen-month-old James Murphy died, the son of Sergeant James Murphy and his wife. He was buried the next day at the post cemetery "in the presence of a large company of sympathizing friends."

Records indicate the child ingested the contents of a bottle of laudanum, an opium derivative. This was available as an over-the-counter patent medicine and was often used for diarrhea, cough, "women's troubles," rheumatic complaints or pain. Laudanum was commonplace in Victorian households, and a bottle of it would last a long time—since only a few drops were needed per dose. Laudanum was sometimes flavored with cinnamon or saffron. The bottle probably had a cork or glass stopper on the top, as this was years before child-proof lids were introduced.

Another baby's death at Fort Davis was that of the son of Lieutenant and Mrs. George A. Dodd on October 17, 1885. Little Allan Dodd was fifteen months old when he died of "cholera infantum," or diarrhea. Back then, there were no IVs to replenish fluids if someone got dehydrated. At the time, Lieutenant Dodd was away from the garrison on detached service in Indian Territory (Oklahoma), and Mrs. Clara Agnes Steele Dodd was at Fort Davis with the baby boy and two daughters—Emily Agnes, four and a half, and

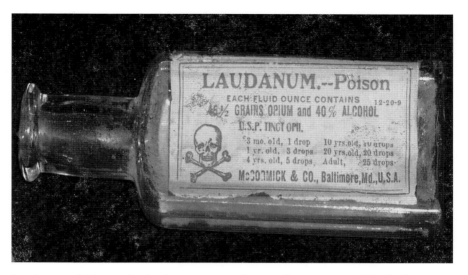

Laudanum, which contained opium, was a popular over-the-counter medicine in the nineteenth century for a variety of ailments. *Author's collection.*

Catherine, three. It must have been heartbreaking for Clara to be separated from her husband and the girls from their father at the time of the baby's death. The child was buried in the Fort Davis Post Cemetery. A little over nine months later, Mrs. Dodd gave birth to another son, Charles, at Fort Sill, and in time, more children—a total of nine—but not all survived childhood. The Dodds lived at army posts all over the American West.

In 1892, the remains of the Murphy child were disinterred and moved to the San Antonio National Cemetery when other Fort Davis bodies—mostly soldiers—were moved there. The body of the Dodd child, however, was not moved, presumably because the grave marker had disappeared and no one knew where the grave was.

Hannah and her husband, Anson Mills, who was a major when he was stationed at Fort Davis from 1882 to 1885, had three children, but only one—their daughter Constance Lydia—survived to adulthood. Their son Anson died at age fifteen of appendicitis in 1894.

In 1872 at Fort Rice, Dakota Territory, an officer's wife named Katherine Garrett Gibson recalled the death of an infant named Fannie. So grieved was she about this death of her friend's baby that she used taffeta and silk from her wedding dress to line the tiny coffin, which a soldier built. The funeral was a simple ceremony. No chaplain was available, she said, so mourners just walked to the cemetery and knelt beside the little grave in prayer. The

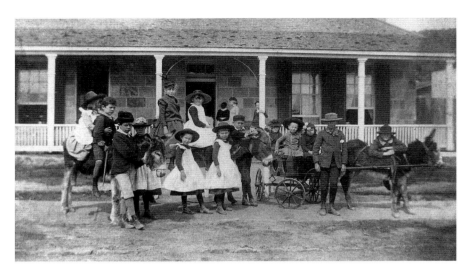

Fort Davis, 1888. As with any military post, children abounded. They lived—and sometimes died. *Fort Davis NHS.*

baby's father was away on field duty at the time, no doubt making it even more difficult for his wife to bear. Fannie was the child of Captain Frederick Benteen and his wife, Catherine "Kate," who had previously buried their other two children as infants. Then, three years later the Benteens buried still another infant at the Fort Rice Post Cemetery. Only one of their five children, Fred, lived to adulthood.

Burying a child is always difficult, but when far from home on the western frontier, it must have been especially so.

Another officer's wife, Ellen McGowan Biddle, who herself lost a child at a remote army fort, wrote about the tremendous heartache—but she also described the way members of the garrison family surrounded the grieving parents with help, support and comfort. Her writings were later published in 1907 in a book entitled *Reminiscences of a Soldier's Wife*. Traveling back east after burying her child on the frontier, Biddle wrote: "I left with one long tender regret, for the grave of my little son under the shadow of the great mountain had to remain."

## *Further Reading*

Biddle, *Reminiscences of a Soldier's Wife*, 195.
Fougera, *With Custer's Cavalry*, 254–56.

# CHAPTER 33

# COCAINE TOOTHACHE DROPS AND OTHER REMEDIES

U ntil there was better understanding of the causes of disease and sickness, doctors in the nineteenth century merely treated symptoms. Some people believed it was better to just stay away from doctors.

Here's a peek inside old medical manuals, textbooks and army records to see common treatments. Some were used by army surgeons or were responses to questions on exams before the Army Medical Board (exam papers are preserved today at the National Archives).

Hint: don't try these "remedies"—they're just to give insight into the past!

SORE THROAT: In 1889, Dr. John Lauderdale sprayed his own sore throat with cocaine mixed with glycerin. In 1868, Dr. Ezra Woodruff suggested poultices of flaxseed and poppy, warm compresses to the throat or various gargles.

CROUP: Treat with antimony (a metallic element), beef essence and wine to drink, ipecac (derived from a root), local applications of warm, moist medicinal compresses or calomel (mercury). If used to excess, calomel, over time, caused a person's hair and teeth to fall out.

HAY FEVER: Cocaine sprayed into the nose was popular in the late nineteenth century when it was found to relieve symptoms, but many denied its addictiveness. Other treatments included arsenic, quinine, iodides and atropia.

TONSILLITIS: A popular 1876 medical manual recommended using ice, quinine (derived from bark of the cinchona tree in South America),

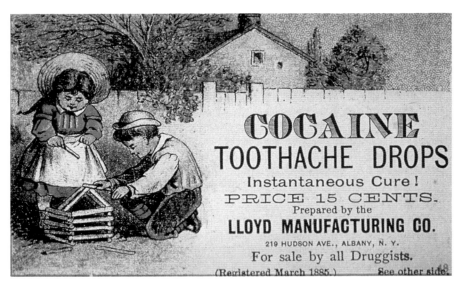

Cocaine toothache drops, 1885. *National Library of Medicine.*

iodides, mercury, guaiac (taken from a tropical tree) or aconite (an herb in the buttercup family known as monkshood, used in traditional medicine to relieve pain). Or there was surgical removal of the tonsils with a tonsillotome. To surgically remove tonsils, the surgeon extended the circular piece with a retractable blade into the throat until it grasped a tonsil, then pulled the "trigger," and the blade guillotined the tonsil. This instrument, made of tempered steel, was stored in a velvet-lined leather case. The cost of a tonsillotome in 1889 was eight to fifteen dollars.

ASTHMA: In 1882, Fort Davis post surgeon Peter R. Egan advised giving injections of morphia or administering large oral doses of whiskey to relax spasms.

PLEURISY, EMPHYSEMA and TB: Dr. Egan recommended giving the patient compressed air or oxygen. Or, to stimulate the central nervous system, administering tonics such as ammonia or strychnine (toxic in high doses; today, strychnine is mainly used in bait, such as rat poison).

SYPHILIS or GONORRHEA: An 1876 medical text listed laudanum enemas; injections of lead, sulphate of zinc or nitrate of silver; medications like morphia, iodides, Dover's Powder, carbolic acid or guaiac; warm dressings to the genitals; lotions to allay the pain; and saltwater baths. Treatment commonly used for soldiers was mercury in the form of calomel liquid or tiny "blue mass pills" or "blue pills" (made of elemental mercury mixed with powdered licorice, rose leaves, honey and sometimes chalk). Mercury was known to be toxic, but it was the best hope for VD in the days before antibiotics. After all, state-of-the-art medical care consisted of treating a powerful disease with a powerful medicine. Consider that we still sometimes treat powerful diseases like cancer with powerful treatments like radiation and chemotherapy.

PNEUMONIA: In 1883, Dr. James E. Pilcher recommended small doses of opiates for restlessness, carbonate of ammonia, stimulants in case of great prostration and for fever: digitalis, arconite or veratrum viride. In some cases—even at this late date in the 1880s, when most physicians had abandoned it—he advised bloodletting/phlebotomy. (Old-timers among us remember seeing the cylindrical pole with diagonal red, white and blue stripes outside barber shops. This was a carryover from bygone days when barbers not only cut hair but also pulled teeth, did minor surgery and performed bloodletting, sometimes using leeches. They were also called barber-surgeons, and the red stripe on their barber poles represented blood—white was for bandages, and blue was for veins!)

DROWNING: Some practitioners recommended tobacco smoke enemas to resuscitate drowning victims. Warmth from the smoke was believed to promote respiration. But most doubted the benefits, leading to the popular saying "blow smoke up one's ass."

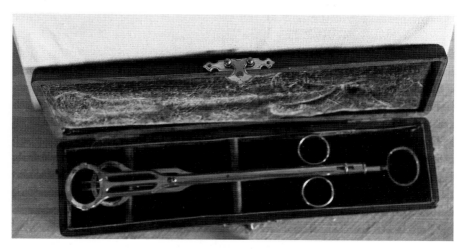

Tonsillotome: insert in throat, stab tonsil, slice, remove—with tonsil. Repeat for second tonsil. *Fort Davis NHS.*

RESPIRATORY AILMENTS: An 1861 military medical manual recommended a mild laxative or hot drink, opium, morphine or over-the-counter Dover's Powder (a mix of opium and ipecac). In 1886, Dr. Paul Clendenin advised alcoholic stimulants (brandy, gin, wine or aromatic spirits of ammonia), turpentine straps on the chest, nutritious food, emetics such as ipecac or alum to induce vomiting and swabbing the throat with lime water or diluted "obleate of mercury."

ACCUMULATION OF FLUID IN LUNGS (EDEMA): Dr. Egan suggested applying dry vacuum cups over the chest and dosing the patient with pilocarpine, digitalis, brandy, ammonia or other stimulants.

CONSTIPATION: Remedies included small doses of rhubarb, castor oil, a pill containing colocynth (from a vine related to watermelon), daily rectal injections of cold water and herbs including taraxacum (dandelion roots) or cascara sagrada (buckhorn tree bark).

INDIGESTION: Arsenic was one of the best tonics, in the opinion of Dr. William Gardner in 1862. Morphine administered by hypodermic injection was what Dr. Lauderdale gave to an officer's wife in 1889.

CHOLERA or CHOLERA MORBUS: Treated with a combination of opium and calomel. Other treatments included enemas of belladonna, laudanum, morphia or black drop (opium and vinegar).

**FACTOID** At Fort Laramie, a hospital attendant devised a treatment to try to deter soldiers from contracting venereal disease—he applied hot or boiling water to the penis. Soldiers went to great lengths to avoid reporting for sick call with symptoms of VD. In the 1880s, the rate of VD in the U.S. Army was about 8 percent—or eighty out of every one thousand men.

## Further Reading

Bartholow, *Practical Treatise on Materia Medica and Therapeutics*, 1876.
Coffman, *Old Army*, 388–89.
Gross, *Manual of Military Surgery* [1861], 127–28.
Lauderdale, "Letterbooks, 1885–1892, Vols. 8–9."
Reimer, communication with author about blue mass pills.
Tiemann, *American Armamentarium Chirurgicum*, 1889.

## CHAPTER 34

# ICE–FOR FEVER, WEDDINGS AND ICE CREAM

I ce played a role in an October 1888 wedding in the Fort Davis post chapel. Private George Freckmann, age twenty-two, married eighteen-year-old Amanda Thompson, stepdaughter of Sergeant Thomas Forsyth. The day before the wedding, hospital steward Jacob Appel preserved a bouquet of white dahlias and roses inside a block of ice—to be presented to the bride on the day of the wedding. Ice was certainly a marvel at the time, and this was surely one of the more unusual wedding gifts the bride received.

Changes in the world were indeed reaching the frontier. In the late 1880s, the army garrison at Fort Davis boasted gaslights outdoors, a telegraph office for speedy communication, a steam-powered pump that filled water storage tanks up on the mountainside to distribute water to outside spigots throughout the fort, proximity to the railroad in both Toyah and Marfa, cameras in the hands of a few people, a personal telephone line that Dr. Lauderdale rigged up from his home on officers' row to the post hospital and an ice machine that produced big blocks of ice.

If ice-making equipment at a nineteenth-century army post seems surprising at a time before electricity, think again. Here's how and why it happened.

In 1887, Fort Davis post commander Colonel Elmer Otis wrote to department headquarters in San Antonio that an ice machine was "deemed essential to the comfort and health of this garrison." A year later, the Army Medical Department issued an ice machine to army posts in Texas for medical purposes. J. Schuehle of San Antonio got a contract to provide six

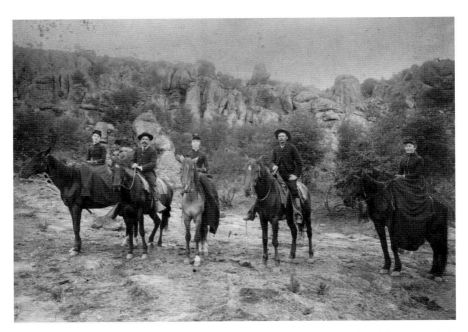

Ice cream may await this daughter and niece of Sergeant Forsyth and other riders upon their return. Women riding sidesaddle wearing corsets and army caps was typical. *Fort Davis NHS.*

ice machines—and one went to the post at Fort Davis. At the time, Texas was a leader in producing artificial ice.

The twofold purpose of the ice machine, according to Fort Davis post surgeon John Lauderdale, was to produce ice for sick members of the post (ice helped control fever) and for the ice machine's steam condenser to provide pure drinking water for the garrison—as army surgeons recognized impure water as a possible source of disease.

When the ice machine arrived at Fort Davis in August 1888, Dr. Lauderdale assumed immediate responsibility for it. Soldiers installed it in the unoccupied band barracks, now Historic Building 24.

In his journal, Dr. Lauderdale often referred to the "ice factory." It involved apparatus such as a boiler with smokestack, ammonia pump, ammonia condenser, pumping engine, freezing tank, grease trap and filter to remove impurities from the creek water being used. Ice was first produced and shared with residents of the garrison on September 22, 1888. Due to various problems, the machinery functioned off and on.

When functional, the machinery used a tremendous amount of wood fuel, which was expensive to obtain. Wood fired the boiler that ran the steam-

**FACTOID** The development of ammonia compression refrigeration in Jefferson, Texas, in 1873 was largely due to the beef industry seeking safe ways to transport beef. Before that, the only way to ship cows was "on the hoof."

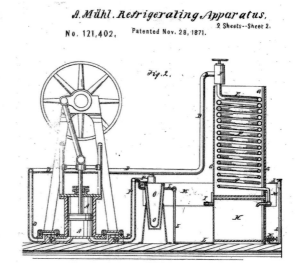

A. Mühl. Refrigerating Apparatus.

No. 121,402. Patented Nov. 28, 1871.

2 Sheets--Sheet 2.

Fig. 2.

Fort Davis had an ice machine for the hospital. Other uses were found for excess ice—like ice cream and frozen flower bouquets. *U.S. Patent and Trademark Office, Andrew Muhl, 1871.*

driven compressor. There were frequent complaints from the quartermaster (QM) about the huge consumption of wood to run the boiler in making ice. Army records reveal rousing controversy between Dr. Lauderdale and the QM over the cost of the wood, which soldiers had to cut in the mountains and haul to the post. Lauderdale claimed the QM charged him for more wood than was actually delivered.

Garrison residents were allowed to purchase ice. Some did so, storing it in an "icebox"—a nonelectric refrigerator that held a block of ice for storing perishable food items. Cork or sawdust was often used as insulation inside icebox doors, which were lined with tin or zinc. A drip pan on the floor under the icebox caught water from the melting ice.

Lauderdale wrote in his journal that an "ice cart went around" the garrison selling ice to residents. He and Colonel Otis discussed how much to charge for the ice. They decided an appropriate cost for fort residents would be ½¢ per pound, and for outsiders, the charge would be four or five times that amount.

On June 3, 1889, fire broke out in the building that housed the ice machine due to a defect in the boiler's flue. The "ice factory" was out of service for three or four weeks. But in August 1889, it produced 990 pounds—or twenty-two large cakes—of ice daily.

For their three-year-old daughter, Marjorie, on September 30, 1889, Dr. Lauderdale and his wife, Josephine, held a birthday party in their home that featured ice cream. What a hit that must have been with the children!

In the making of ice, ammonia—the refrigerant—is put under compression—and it is flammable. Strong winds carried off the "ice factory" roof in March 1890, but it was soon operating again. Then the unthinkable happened: the ice machine building caught fire and was completely destroyed. Never again was ice made at the garrison. That was surely a disappointment.

The Lauderdales left Fort Davis in May 1890 to move to Fort Ontario, New York. It had been an adventure with the ice machine at Fort Davis, with mechanical frustrations and satisfying moments, too. Dr. Lauderdale's journals provide insight into some of the challenges of life on the western frontier—eased just a bit by amenities like ice and even ice cream.

## Further Reading

Fort Davis National Historic Site archival library.
Greene, *Historic Resource Study: Fort Davis*, 151.
Lauderdale, "Letterbooks, 1885–1892, Vols. 8–9."

## CHAPTER 35

# SCALPS AND SKULLS

**M**any people are not aware of how ruthlessly Native peoples were nearly hunted to extinction through the scalp-buying process, especially in Mexico but apparently in California, too, after the Gold Rush.

In Mexico, the reward given by the Mexican government for an "Indian" scalp might be $100 or $150—even up to $250 for the scalp of an "Indian" woman! (That was a lot of money—$150 in 1850 would be worth almost $5,000 today.)

One notorious and unscrupulous scalp hunter with a violent past in the American Southwest, Joel "John" Glanton from South Carolina, even killed and scalped Mexican people then turned them in as "Indian" scalps! Driven by greed, Glanton and his gang were known to kill and scalp peaceful farming "Indian" people to turn in their scalps for a reward. Glanton, who operated around the southwestern United States and northern Mexico, died in 1850 in Arizona at the hands of "Indians," probably Yuma or Quechan. Some reports say he was scalped.

Another contemptible mercenary scalp hunter was James Kirker, born in Ireland. In one year, he reportedly collected $100,000 for scalps—and that was a lot of money in the mid-1800s. Stories vary about Kirker, whose life was at times colorful but treacherous. He died in 1852.

Here's a horrid story to make scalp-hunting a little more personal. In the mid-1850s, an older Mescalero Apache chief named Huero Garanza befriended the U.S. Army and visited the Fort Davis garrison. The army was interested in hiring him as a guide. While Chief Garanza was there, post surgeon Andrew Jackson Foard walked to a hospital closet to show Garanza the doctor's skull collection. But Garanza refused to look at the skulls, communicating to the physician that it was "bad medicine" to do so. Not long afterward, an angry rancher from Presidio del Norte who had lost cattle to "Indian" depredations hired a posse of Mexicans. They ambushed and killed Chief Garanza and three Lipans who were with him. Bliss felt Garanza was a good man and wrote in his journal that he sincerely hoped Garanza's skull was not exchanged for bounty money or sold to the Mexican government.

It is important to note that U.S. Army doctors on the frontier did autopsies after soldiers died in order to learn more about disease and injury. As stated in chapter 15, U.S. Army physicians at far-flung garrisons were directed to send "unusual specimens" of medical interest (such as lungs, kidneys, etc.) to the Army Medical Museum in Washington, D.C., to be used as teaching tools. The Army Medical Museum surely received a lot of skulls, as well as other body parts, from frontier army doctors. Today, the museum has over five thousand skeletal specimens and more than twenty-five million bones, organs and other intriguing, sometimes grim, items—including brains! Next time you're near Washington, D.C., don't miss it—now called the National Museum of Health and Medicine, it's free!

There was also an eagerness to learn about animals and plants on the frontier. In March 1870, Fort Davis post surgeon Daniel Weisel received notice to collect and ship mammal skeletons to the Army Medical Museum. Dr. Weisel forwarded the message to the post adjutant to solicit the help of soldiers in the field to collect mammal skeletons.

It is not clear why, in the 1850s, post surgeon Andrew J. Foard had a skull collection at the Fort Davis post hospital. It is likely his curiosity to learn was the driving factor.

**FACTOID** The skull of at least one soldier who died at Fort Davis was shipped to the Army Medical Museum for study: that of Corporal Richard Robinson, in 1878. (See chapter 15.) A theory prevailed then that the size of a person's head determined intelligence—so there was curiosity about comparing skulls of White, Black and Native peoples, as well as of women and men. There was a commonly held theory in the nineteenth century that women's heads were smaller and thus they were intellectually inferior to men!

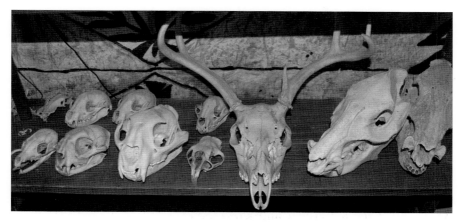

Mammal skull collection from the Fort Davis area, probably similar to Dr. Weisel's own collection: javelina, deer, porcupine, mountain lion, bobcat, fox, raccoon. *Author's collection.*

Nor is it known whether his collection contained human skulls, or animal skulls—or both. This was before 1862 when the U.S. Army's surgeon general first asked physicians to send specimens to the army nurses for research purposes.

## *Further Reading*

Clary, "Role of the Army Surgeon [...] Daniel Weisel," 64.
Greene, *Historic Resource Study: Fort Davis*, 67, 126–28.
Smith, *Borderlander*, 226.
Thrapp, *Encyclopedia of Frontier Biography*, vol. 2, 564.

## CHAPTER 36

# NO TALKING AFTER BEDTIME, 8½ P.M.

## Army Hospital Rules

**W**alking through an old nineteenth-century army hospital today, you can almost smell rotting, gangrenous flesh. When the wind blows eerily through creaking roof timbers, it's as if good spirits of patients long dead are calling out a haunting greeting.

Imagine for a moment what it might have been like to be a patient in the 1800s. To give some idea of the atmosphere, here's a set of rules that the U.S. Army's 1862 *Hospital Steward's Manual,* written by Dr. J.J. Woodward, recommended be displayed on the walls of army hospital wards:

*No smoking, swearing, loud talking, or spitting on the floor…and no defacing of the building in any way.*

*Patients must make their beds every morning, if able.*

*Patients must undress before occupying a hospital bed.*

*Patients must take a bath upon admission to the hospital, wash face & hands daily, and keep their bodies clean—attendants will help if needed.*

*Patients and nurses must be present when Surgeon visits the ward and, if able, must stand when he enters.*

*No talking after bedtime, 8 ½ P. M.*

*Lights are lowered in the ward at 9 P. M. and other hospital lights are extinguished at Taps.*

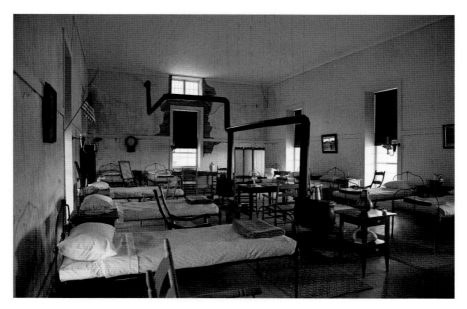

Restored north ward at Fort Davis post hospital. *Fort Davis NHS.*

> *Patients and nurses are forbidden to enter the Office or Kitchen or to lounge about the halls.*
>
> *No one is allowed to enter the hospital without permission from the Doctor.*
>
> *No spiritous liquors or provisions may be brought by patients' friends or relatives into the hospital without permission.*
>
> *Infractions such as drunkenness, disorderly conduct, or disobedience to orders will be punished.*

# Further Reading

Woodward, *Hospital Steward's Manual* [1862], 95–97.

## CHAPTER 37

# FEMALE ARMY SURGEON RECEIVES MEDAL OF HONOR

**N**one of the physicians hired by the U.S. Army Medical Department during the nineteenth century were women. To be an army surgeon, one had to be a male, age twenty-two to twenty-eight, a citizen by birth or naturalization and a graduate of a "regular" or allopathic medical college.

Here's the story, however, of a woman—Mary Edwards Walker, MD, of New York—who graduated from medical school in 1855 and later worked as a contract surgeon for the Union army during the Civil War.

Dr. Walker graduated with honors with an MD from Syracuse Medical College, the only woman in the graduating class. She was one of a small number of female doctors in America at the time, the first being British-born Dr. Elizabeth Blackwell, who graduated from Geneva Medical College in New York in 1849. After graduation, Dr. Walker had a difficult time attracting patients to her medical practice because of the mistrust of female doctors at the time.

At the outbreak of the Civil War, she tried to get a job with the Army Medical Department but was rejected because she was female. The Union army allowed her to work as a nurse and, in 1863, employed her as a civilian physician.

In 1865, Dr. Walker was thirty-three years old when President Andrew Johnson presented her with the Medal of Honor. Two generals, including William Tecumseh Sherman, had nominated her for the medal.

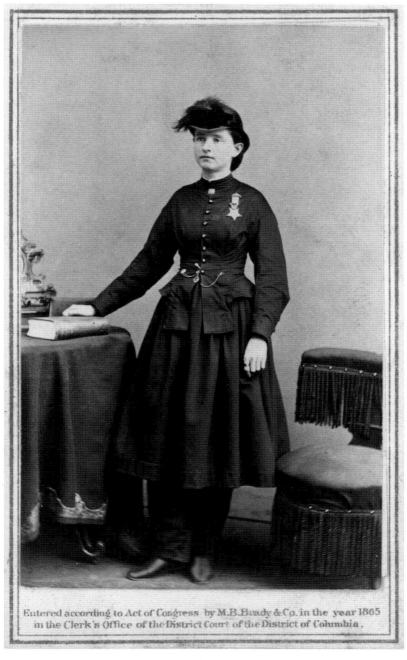

Entered according to Act of Congress by M.B. Brady & Co. in the year 1865
in the Clerk's Office of the District Court of the District of Columbia.

Dr. Mary Edwards Walker wearing the Medal of Honor—and trousers under her skirt. *Library of Congress.*

Her courageous action earning her this prestigious award took place the previous year when she was working for the Union army as a contract surgeon. Ignoring the danger to herself, she rendered medical treatment to injured soldiers. She even crossed enemy lines to do so, and when captured as a spy, she was imprisoned as a prisoner of war at Richmond for four months until she was exchanged for a Confederate physician.

According to the presidential order that awarded Dr. Walker the Medal of Honor for Meritorious Service, she had "devoted herself with much patriotic zeal to the sick and wounded soldiers, both in the field and hospitals, to the detriment of her own health, and has also endured hardships as a prisoner-of-war four months in a Southern prison."

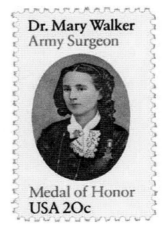

Postage stamp issued in 1982 by the U.S. Postal Service depicting Dr. Mary Walker. *Author's collection.*

Walker worked for other causes of the day, including the suffrage, antislavery and temperance movements. In 1871, she published a book of essays on women's rights titled *Hit.* She also advocated for lawmakers to give pensions to female army nurses—which they finally did in 1892, twenty-seven years after the Civil War ended. (See Chapter 5 for the ANPA, which had stipulations and was limited to nurses in the Union army only.)

More sensible clothing for women was another cause for which Walker advocated. She wrote that corsets were physically damaging and that stockings held up with elastic or other bands impeded circulation and caused varicose veins. She ridiculed as absurd the practice of some women having both little toes removed in order to wear smaller shoes. She felt such fashions predisposed women to diseases, nervousness and debility—taxing the nerves, brain, blood vessels and spinal column and draining women of vitality.

Walker wore modified clothing herself, including trousers. Other women were adopting the style of long pants called "pantalettes" or "bloomers" under a knee-length dress—a style known one hundred years later as the pantsuit. When criticized for wearing what was considered then to be men's clothing, she remarked, "I don't wear men's clothes—I wear my own clothes!"

In 1917, two years before her death at age eighty-six, the army rescinded her Medal of Honor along with those of 910 other noncombatants when

> **FACTOID** Other women doctors in nineteenth-century America
> included Dr. Chloe Annette Buckel, Dr. Oriana Moon Andrews, Dr.
> Esther Hill Hawks, Dr. Sarah Ann Chadwick Clapp, Dr. Mary Frame
> Thomas, Dr. Rebecca Davis Lee Crumpler, Dr. Elizabeth Blackwell,
> Dr. Emily Blackwell, Dr. Marie Zakrzewska and Dr. Susan La Flesche
> Picotte (the first Indigenous woman to receive a medical degree in
> the United States, she graduated in 1889 from the Women's Medical
> College of Pennsylvania).

eligibility requirements changed. History tells us that she complained, refused to return her Medal of Honor and continued to wear it until her death.

Years later, Walker's great-niece pressed the issue of restoring her aunt's Medal of Honor, even taking it to the White House. Finally, in 1977, President Jimmy Carter reinstated her Medal of Honor. Of the over 3,500 recipients to date, Dr. Mary Edwards Walker is the only woman so far to receive the Medal of Honor.

## Further Reading

Blanton and Cook, *They Fought Like Demons: Women Soldiers in the Civil War*, 96.
Coe, "Mary Walker's Quest to be Appointed as a Union Doctor in the Civil War."
Graf, *Woman of Honor: Dr. Mary E. Walker*.
Lineberry, "I Wear My Own Clothes."
National Park Service, "Dr. Mary Edwards Walker."
*New York Times*, obituary of Dr. Mary Edwards Walker.
Oswego State University of New York, Biography of Dr. Mary Edwards Walker.
Walker, Medal of Honor, 1974–77.
Wright, biographical paper on Dr. Mary Walker.

## CHAPTER 38

# DYING TOO YOUNG

Annie M. Sullivan Nolan died at Fort Concho, Texas, in February 1877. She was only twenty-nine. "Quick consumption" is how another officer's wife described her terminal illness—tuberculosis. Born in New York, Annie was the wife of Captain Nicholas Merritt Nolan, Tenth U.S. Cavalry.

At the time of Annie's death, she and Nicholas had two children: ten-year-old Katie (Katherine Agatha) and six-year-old Ned (Edmond Merritt). Katie was attending school two hundred miles away in San Antonio at the Ursuline Convent.

Annie was embalmed and placed in a "fine coffin" built just for her. Then Captain Nolan accompanied the body of his beloved wife from Fort Concho for burial in the San Antonio National Cemetery.

A year and a half later, in August 1878, Captain Nolan married nineteen-year-old Anne Eleanor Dwyer. Their daughter, Elizabeth, was born at Fort Davis when Nolan was stationed there. Anne's sister, Mollie Dwyer, is entwined in the story of Lieutenant Henry O. Flipper, the U.S. Army's first African American officer.

In December 1882, Nolan was promoted to major and transferred from the Tenth Cavalry to the Third Cavalry. Six months later, the army placed him in command of Fort Huachuca, Arizona Territory. Not long afterwards, Nolan died. Cause of death was "brain consumption" or "apoplexy"—probably a stroke. He was forty-eight. Anne Eleanor, his second wife, was twenty-four.

Western Union telegram sent October 27, 1883, to the adjutant general, notifying him of Major Nolan's death. *Fort Larned NHS website, National Archives.*

When Major Nolan died in October 1883, he was traveling with a detachment of cavalry from Fort Apache to the new town of Holbrook in Navajo County. There, he planned to meet his family to begin two weeks' leave. Telegram notification about Major Nolan's death was sent to the adjutant general in Washington, D.C., from Fort Wingate, New Mexico Territory, two days after Nolan died. It indicates the army planned to bury him at Fort Wingate. Later sources indicate his body was embalmed and shipped for burial in San Antonio National Cemetery, where his first wife was buried. Nicholas Nolan had served in the U.S. Army for over thirty years, since he first came to America from Ireland in 1852, at age seventeen.

Anne/Annie E. Dwyer Nolan returned to civilian life and applied for a widow's pension, including an allotment for their young daughter, Elizabeth, just a toddler then, as well as for Nolan's son Ned (thirteen) by his first wife. By that time, his daughter Katie was seventeen or eighteen—too old for a parent or guardian to receive a pension allowance for her.

Anne died in 1907 in her late forties and is buried at Arlington Cemetery. Her gravestone bears her maiden name. She and Nicholas Nolan were only married for three years when he died. Lots of frontier army stories seem to end like this, with individuals dying too young. Medical science still had a long way to go.

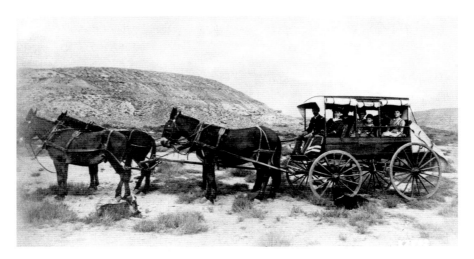

Officer and his family riding in army ambulance—accompanied by their dogs. Officers sometimes used army ambulances as personal conveyances. *Western History Collection, University of Oklahoma Libraries.*

Another very sick officer's wife on the western frontier was Alice Beverly Potter Andrews. She was the wife of Colonel George Lippitt Andrews, commanding officer at Fort Davis in the early 1870s. He requested and was granted leave to travel with her back east, where she was to have surgery.

Their five-hundred-plus-mile ride across Texas in an army ambulance was dreadful for her; this was a decade before the railroad came to west Texas. Alice died at age forty-six on April 29, 1873, soon after they reached New York—eight weeks after leaving Fort Davis. She was buried near her family home in Providence, Rhode Island, and later moved to Arlington Cemetery.

The next year, Colonel Andrews married a widow, Emily Kemble Oliver Brown, in Maine. She was thirty-nine, and he was forty-six. He had a fulfilling army career and needed a wife to make his life complete.

Emily recorded the cross-country part of their journey from Austin to Fort Davis in diary form as letters written to her father back east. Travel time—August 11 to September 8, 1874—was four weeks, minus a week's layover at Fort Stockton. Today, a car trip from Austin to Fort Davis takes seven or eight hours. Here's the opening of her first letter:

> *My Dearest Father,*
> *Feeling sure that some little account of our trip through Texas would be entertaining to you, I have tried to note down each days doings, and herewith send them to you. Necessarily this has often been written in the greatest*

*hurry, either when just ready for a start in the morning, or when tired and sleepy after a long days march, so you must read with the greatest leniency.*

With Emily was her teenage daughter, Matilda "Maud" Brown, from her first marriage. The Andrews' escort for the journey across Texas was a group of Twenty-Fifth Infantry soldiers. Being hauled along with them was Emily's beloved piano, which came by ship from Boston to Galveston.

The escort included thirteen soldiers, four six-mule teams, four mules to pull the army ambulance (a light wagon equipped with springs and removable leather seats) for Emily and Maud, as well as other "necessary equipage." Colonel Andrews rode his favorite horse, Billy. At night, Emily described sleeping on beds with horsehair mattresses in a tent that was fourteen feet square and had a tarpaulin floor covering. What an ordeal—yet such luxury.

Imagine traveling in a wagon during the 1870s: flooding rivers to cross, no air-conditioning, no running water or flush toilets, no cell phones or electronic devices—and there were days when "Indians" were spotted nearby, a big cause for concern. If only there were letters written by Native peoples, comparable to Emily's. One wonders what they thought about the increasing amount of traffic and settlers encroaching on their lands.

## Further Reading

Hooker, *Child of the Fighting Tenth: On the Frontier with the Buffalo Soldiers.*

Leckie, *The Colonel's Lady on the Western Frontier: The Correspondence of Alice Kirk Grierson*, 94–95.

Myres, "A Woman's View of the Texas Frontier, 1874: Diary of Emily K. Andrews."

Smith, Thompson, Wooster and Pingenot, *Reminiscences of Major General Zenas R. Bliss*, 465.

# CHAPTER 39

# WHAT WOULD YOU NAME
# YOUR HORSE?

Horses were an integral part of life in the nineteenth-century army. Cavalry regiments served at garrisons all over the West, and a trooper took excellent care of his horse—because in some situations, he depended on his horse for survival. Before daily "mess call"

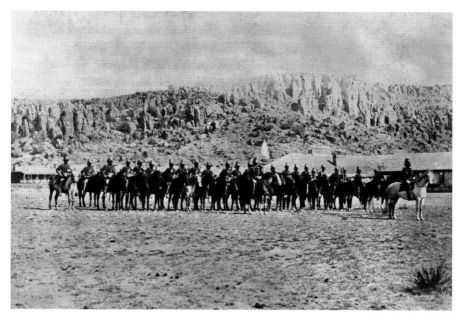

*Opposite*: Horses of Ninth Cavalry, Troop H at Fort Bliss, Texas, July 1871. List gives each horse's name, age, size, color, how/when acquired, length in service, rider's name and rank. *Fort Davis NHS.*

*Above*: Ninth U.S. Cavalry troopers in dress uniform, Fort Davis, 1875. *Fort Davis NHS.*

for his own breakfast, a cavalryman went to the stables to feed and care for his horse.

At Fort Davis in January 1885, Lieutenant John Bigelow, Tenth U.S. Cavalry, wrote in his journal that he attended two veterinary lectures per week with the men, as well as a weekly class at the stables. At one class, they dissected a horse. The veterinary surgeon at the time was Dr. A.E. Buzard, who was a civilian veterinarian under contract with the army to care for horses and train farriers.

A veterinary surgeon was typically stationed at posts designated as regimental headquarters. In 1870, Dr. Leuther Sargent was Ninth U.S. Cavalry veterinary surgeon at Fort Davis, which was regimental headquarters at the time. The 1870 census says Sargent was forty-six, a native of Vermont and living at the garrison with his wife, Alcaria, thirty, born in Mexico, and two children, owning personal property valued at $150.

**FACTOID** Lieutenant John Bigelow faithfully kept a journal, giving insight into life at frontier army posts. In 1884, he wrote that Fort Davis commanding officer Colonel Benjamin Grierson traveled home to Illinois in order to vote in the U.S. presidential election. During the Civil War, some states had allowed absentee voting for those away from home due to military service. After the Civil War, absentee voting was not formally addressed by Congress until 1932, although in 1918, some state legislatures passed a temporary absentee voting law for World War I soldiers.

Cavalry soldiers often gave their horses interesting names. In an actual 1871 listing of horses of some Ninth U.S. Cavalry troopers at Fort Bliss, Texas, you can see names like Eagle, Spitfire, Apache, Eclipse, Ant Eater, Old Nick, Hercules, Sphinx and Thunder.

## Further Reading

Bigelow, *Garrison Tangles in the Friendless Tenth*, 44.

CHAPTER 40

# WHAT DID THEY CALL PTSD?

ivine madness" is what ancient Greeks called it. Some nineteenth-century doctors labeled it "melancholia." During the American Civil War, it was known as "soldier's heart" or "nostalgia." In World War I, they called it "shell shock" and in World War II, "combat fatigue" or "battle fatigue."

These were some of the terms for various symptoms believed to be due to anxiety, despair or even homesickness that at times rendered soldiers unable to function normally. It was not understood how trauma from war or the insane chaos of being in battle impacted the human psyche.

Here's an 1878 medical account of a young African American soldier who was hospitalized after being stationed at an isolated Fort Davis outpost and was hallucinating. He was a guard at a stage stop near a waterhole that the Apaches frequented. The army surgeon, who diagnosed the condition as "melancholia," wrote:

> *Private W.H. Anderson, Co. I, 25th Infantry, was admitted into Post Hospital on April 4, 1878, suffering with hallucinations being in a state of terror for fear of indians and citizens. He has been on duty as stage station guard at Eagle Springs, Tex., and the sergeant in command of guard was compelled to disarm him and place him under restraint while sending him back to Fort Davis, Tex.*

Unfortunately, no known letters exist to tell the story from Private Anderson's perspective, but with Apaches freely roaming the area at the

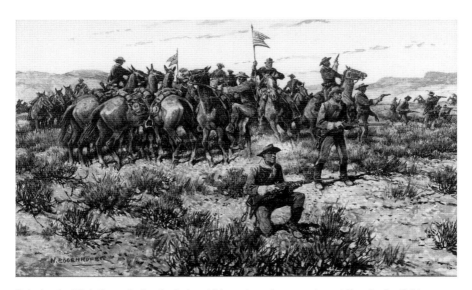

Painting by Nick Eggenhofer depicting African American cavalry soldiers in the field engaging Apaches. *Display at Fort Davis NHS museum.*

time, it is understandable that as a guard who spent hours alone protecting a very remote stage stop, he would have been afraid. He was also a Black man, likely frightened for his life because of people who might see him as a threat at a time when lynchings of Blacks were common occurrences in some parts of America. Who knows what previous experiences Private Anderson might have had to make him fearful of "indians and citizens."

In 1877, another soldier, this time at Fort Abraham Lincoln, Dakota Territory, was brought in to the post hospital after a battle with Nez Perce. The army medical report says he "almost constantly talked about Indians and after he had tried to insert the tines of a fork in an ear to dog Indians out, he was placed in a strait jacket."

**FACTOID** Per U.S. Army records, Company K of the Tenth U.S. Cavalry traveled 3,500 miles in two months, October and November 1880, while patrolling west Texas, searching for Apaches. That's a lot of miles on horseback, averaging fifty-seven miles per day. It was an unsettled time—Apache leader Victorio and his followers, including women and children, who were being pursued by the military, retreated to Mexico to seek refuge. There, Victorio, his warriors and some Apache women were killed by Mexican soldiers at Tres Castillos on October 14, 1880. Apache tradition maintains that Victorio fell on his own knife rather than be killed by Mexican soldiers. In the aftermath, sixty-eight Apache women and children were taken captive and were reportedly "assimilated" into Mexican families. Nobody wins in war—both sides lose.

**FACTOID** At sunrise on October 26, 1880, "about 30 Indians" attacked fourteen soldiers in camp who were guarding a remote spring-fed waterhole at Hot Springs/Ojo Caliente, not far from the Mexican border, sixty to seventy miles southwest of Fort Davis. Chaos ensued, five of the soldiers were killed and "the rest of the men became demoralized and scattered to make their escape by running away, abandoning most of their clothing, arms, horses, equipments, etc. which were captured by the Indians." Two of the dead men's bodies were "badly mutilated," having twenty-inch-long picket pins driven through them into the ground. The dead Tenth Cavalry troopers, all Black, were later buried at the scene. Two soldiers were reported as missing in action—but a year later, one of those men showed up in the army records as being discharged for disability, and the other soldier was apprehended over three years later as a deserter.

At times, a soldier whose behavior was abnormal and inexplicably bizarre was sent to the government's "Asylum for the Insane" in Washington, D.C. One army doctor who was sent there as a patient in the spring of 1889 was Dr. Henry Sutton Tarring Harris, whose diagnosis was "acute insanity—melancholia with delusions." Another physician believed Dr. Harris's problem was alcohol addiction or alcoholism, which was sometimes blamed for stress from war-related incidents. Sometimes a soldier was sent to Alcatraz Island (a facility for military prisoners) in San Francisco Bay for what might have been neurological issues related to trauma like being under attack by what army reports usually called "Indians."

Late in the twentieth century—well after the Vietnam War—America finally began to recognize post-traumatic stress disorder, or PTSD, as something that adversely affects soldiers and veterans, as well as people who have experienced stressful events such as tsunamis, earthquakes, hurricanes, sexual trauma, terrorist experiences or traumatic brain injuries.

We know now that some of the worst injuries from war-related activities occur to the psyche—defined variously as the mind, the brain, the soul or the spirit.

## Further Reading

Lauderdale, "Letterbooks, 1885–1892, vol. 8–9."
Mulford, *Fighting Indians!*, 133.
Rickey, *Forty Miles a Day on Beans and Hay*, 329.
U.S. Army, Medical History of Posts: Fort Davis 1868–1891.

# CHAPTER 41

# CEMETERIES

## Fort Davis, Where Are Your Dead?

A graveyard, with its eerie silence, brings to mind our mortality. There, all humanity is reduced to a common denominator: death—the one truth we all face.

During the thirty-two years that Fort Davis was an active army post, from 1854 to 1891, the garrison used five different post cemetery locations at various times. One was off-post, and one locale at the fort was used during two distinct time periods.

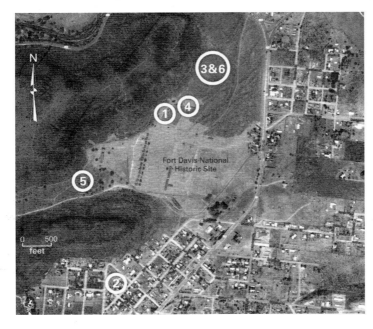

Locations of Fort Davis post cemeteries, 1854–91. *Fort Davis NHS.*

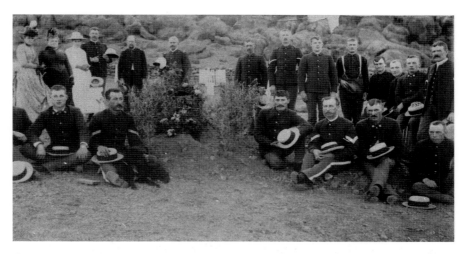

Only known photo at Fort Davis Post Cemetery. It shows soldiers, officers and wives on Decoration Day, Thursday, May 30, 1889. *Lauderdale, Yale University, Beinecke Library.*

**FACTOID** On Wednesday, May 29, 1889, post surgeon J.V. Lauderdale wrote in his journal: "Tomorrow is Decoration Day, but the earth is so dry that I do not know where the flowers will come from wherewith to decorate the graves of our dead soldiers." The name was later changed from Decoration Day to Memorial Day. Traditionally, it was observed on May 30 but nowadays, on the last Monday in May. The tradition of decorating the graves of fallen soldiers began in the United States around the time of the Civil War, following the practice of ancient Greeks and Romans to honor their fallen.

The quartermaster cared for the post cemetery, but apparently the job he did was not always satisfactory. In May 1876, post chaplain George G. Mullins wrote in a report that "the graves of the U.S. soldiers at this Post are in sad state of neglect." In the mid-1880s, Lieutenant John Bigelow noted in his journal how busy post quartermaster Captain Mason M. Maxon was tending his real estate endeavors in the local area: i.e., his stock of hundreds of Angora goats on nearby leased land.

When the U.S. Army deactivated Fort Davis in June 1891, the property reverted to John James, the owner who leased it to the federal government. Early the next year, a west Texas local named David Merrill obtained a government contract to disinter bodies from marked graves at the final post cemetery. He and his son Jesse moved the bodies with their grave markers for rail shipment from Marfa to the

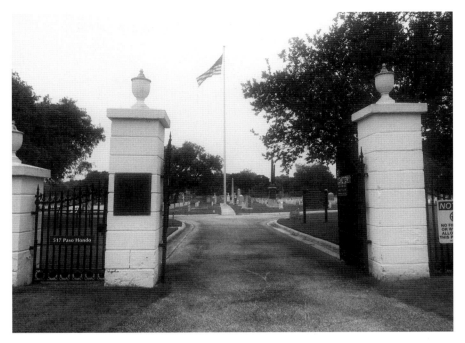

Entrance to San Antonio National Cemetery. Many Fort Davis dead were reinterred there after the army closed the garrison. *Photo by author.*

**FACTOID** 169 soldiers died while assigned to Fort Davis from 1854 to 1891. Of these, research shows that twenty-one were killed by "Indians"—about 13 percent of all deaths.

Disease: 105 (over 60 percent)
Accidents: 26
Murdered (defined as "malicious killings"): 8
Homicides (defined as "justifiable killings"): 2
Suicides: 3
KIA: 13
MIA: 12

San Antonio National Cemetery. Later, all the original grave markers from Fort Davis burials were replaced with uniform white headstones.

Of the 209 military and civilian deaths associated with the Fort Davis garrison, burial locations of 112 are known—most at San Antonio National Cemetery. That leaves 97 bodies unaccounted for today, including 31 lost in the field, as well as 49 soldiers and 11 civilians likely still buried somewhere at Fort Davis.

**FACTOID** The national cemetery system was begun in 1862 for Civil War dead. That year, there were 14 national cemeteries; ten years later, there were 74. The Department of Veterans Affairs now maintains 142 national cemeteries in 40 states, as well as 33 soldiers' lots and monument sites.

## Further Reading

Bigelow, *Garrison Tangles in the Friendless Tenth*, 15.
Deglman and Smith, "Roll Call of the Dead," 43–66.
Greene, *Historic Resource Study: Fort Davis*, 291–95.
Williams, "Care of the Dead," 2–3.

**CHAPTER 42**

# SCURVY

## A Monstrous and Wicked Disease for Soldiers, Sailors and Pirates

Three Ninth Cavalry soldiers died from scurvy at Fort Davis in 1868: Privates David Johnson, William Asberry and Joseph Taylor. They were Black troopers, probably coming out of slavery—so they likely came into the military malnourished and physically weak.

Serious problems with scurvy plagued the U.S. Army for decades in the 1800s, even when the British navy knew better. For years, according to army historian Mary C. Gillett, the army erroneously—and stubbornly—believed that scurvy was caused by factors like dampness, fatigue, anxiety or excessive salt. In fact, before the Civil War, scurvy in the army was a common disease.

Scurvy is a debilitating nutritional deficiency disease. A staggering two million sailors died around the world from scurvy during what is known as the Age of Discovery, from 1500 to the mid-1800s. Rations aboard those old sailing ships were basics like salted meat, hard bread full of weevils, beer and rum—altogether bland and monotonous, and devoid

**FACTOID** Scurvy is a horrible way to die. In the early stage, a person feels tired and has aching joints and leg muscles. The gums swell, itch and feel hot. Ulcers and gangrene develop on the skin. Swollen gums start to rot, bleed and smell like decaying flesh. Teeth become loose. The breath becomes foul. Legs swell. Bones, muscles and joints are excruciatingly painful. Finally, high fever develops, black spots appear on the skin, fits of fainting and trembling occur and there is gasping for breath and, finally, death—caused by hemorrhaging in the heart and brain.

of fresh fruits and vegetables. Some historians believe that scurvy killed more seafarers than shipwrecks, foul weather, battles, pirates and all other diseases combined! (Blackbeard was killed in 1718 in his thirties! If he had lived longer, maybe he might have been a victim of scurvy.)

Oddly enough, through the centuries, humans have known about preventatives for scurvy, but those were either lost and rediscovered or were considered too impracticable to be implemented. It wasn't just sailors who died of scurvy; soldiers in the U.S. Army did too.

For soldiers stationed at remote army posts in the nineteenth century before the days of refrigeration, the challenge was how to ship oranges, lemons or limes and then to provide long-term storage for the citrus fruit. Just try to keep an orange at room temperature for three to six months and see how it tastes.

Supply wagons moved very slowly, especially when pulled by oxen. In the 1870s, an army supply wagon train carrying "bacon" left San Antonio in February and did not arrive at Fort Davis until April. The trip took seventy-one days. (Today, that trip of about four hundred miles would take about six hours in a car.) Imagine what that bacon—oozing with fat—must have looked and smelled like after being in unrefrigerated wagons for ten weeks! Well, the late arrival "ruffled some feathers" indeed. The assistant quartermaster complained vehemently that it would have taken only fifty-three days if the wagons had been pulled by mules instead of oxen. When the wagon train straggled into Fort Davis, much of the bacon was spoiled, but luckily it was able to be sold at auction to locals to recoup some of the financial loss to the government. Sold at auction?? Hmm, perhaps it was purchased for making soap.

Soldiers' diet on the frontier consisted of little in the way of fresh food. A standard army ration was bread, coffee, beans and occasionally a little meat. No wonder soldiers' bodies suffered under the strain of a physically demanding lifestyle! Take a look at historic photos of army enlisted men—being overweight was not an issue.

**FACTOID** In the mid-1700s, James Lind, a Scottish physician working for the Royal Navy, theorized that citrus fruit counteracted scurvy. At first, he was ridiculed for such a preposterous idea, but when citrus fruit was given to sailors aboard British Navy ships and it helped prevent scurvy, the idea caught on. At the time, the words "lemon" and "lime" were used interchangeably, and British sailors began to be called "limeys" because, by the end of the century, the Royal Navy added citrus juice to sailors' daily rations of "grog" (watered-down rum) to prevent scurvy. It worked—deaths from scurvy dropped precipitously.

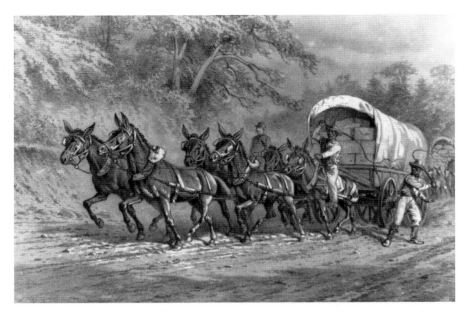

Supply trains moved slowly when pulled by mules or horses—even more slowly when pulled by oxen. Railroads would change that. *Library of Congress*.

Following the Civil War, the U.S. Army Medical Department began encouraging troopers at remote garrisons to grow gardens and to hunt for fresh meat to supplement the ration. Perhaps the deaths of the three Fort Davis troopers due to scurvy in 1868 were a major factor causing post surgeon Daniel Weisel to advocate for soldiers to plant vegetable gardens. Research into the Army Medical Department's *Registers of the Sick and Wounded* shows that in the decade 1880–1889 at Fort Davis, after vegetables were added to rations, doctors reported no deaths from scurvy and only two cases of it, both in 1880.

Nobody had heard of vitamins then, so vitamin C was not a household word. It was acknowledged at the time, however, that fresh fruits and vegetables were the preventative—aided by vinegar, fresh onions and potatoes. In the field, a soldier's ration might include an onion (which has a modicum of vitamin C) kept in a sock!

## *Further Reading*

Gillett, *Army Medical Department*, 14–18.
Sobel, *Longitude: The Story of a Lone Genius*, 14.
U.S. Army, Medical Records, Fort Davis.

## CHAPTER 43

# DIED OF SOFTENING OF THE BRAIN

G enerally, the army did not admit civilians to the post hospital. In cases of dire necessity, however, the army provided medical care for discharged soldiers at frontier garrisons when they remained in the vicinity of their discharge from the army. The Fort Davis medical records reveal that at least twice, the post hospital admitted an ex-soldier.

One was John McCann, a former private in the Third U.S. Cavalry who had been discharged for disability. According to the death record, he was a civilian when he died in the post hospital from "chronic dysentery" on September 11, 1885. He was buried the next day in the post cemetery, in grave number 83. He was twenty-four years old.

"Softening of the brain" was the diagnosis listed for another ex-soldier, John H. Mason, an "indigent citizen" who died at the Fort Davis post hospital in June 1886 after a hospital stay of fourteen months. Here's his story.

Mason was a former corporal in the Tenth U.S. Cavalry, discharged for disability eighteen months earlier in October 1884. At the time of his discharge, Mason's character rating was "excellent," and he had served eleven years in the army. Six months after Mason's discharge, the post commander at Fort Davis instructed the surgeon to admit him to the hospital "as a necessary act of humanity." According to the reports, Mason—who was forty-three—was "indigent, sick, and feeble-minded" and had no other means of caring for himself.

The post hospital admitted ex-corporal Mason, and he was still there a year later when the board of commissioners at the Old Soldiers' Home in Washington, D.C., agreed to pay the army at Fort Davis eight dollars per

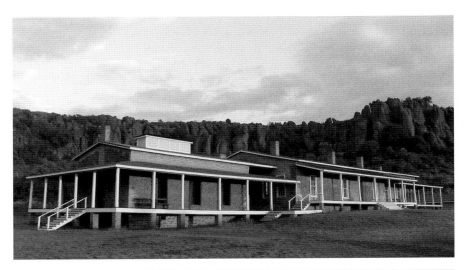

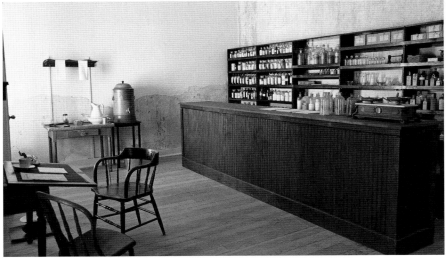

*Top*: Fort Davis post hospital as it appears today. *Photo by Max Kandler.*

*Bottom*: Dispensary, recently restored, at the Fort Davis post hospital. *Fort Davis NHS.*

month for Mason's care, retroactive to May 1885. The next year, on June 11, 1886, the secretary of war directed eighty cents per day to be paid by the Old Soldiers' Home to continue Mason's care at the Fort Davis post hospital, but Mason died nine days later, on June 20, in the post hospital.

Cause of death was "softening of the brain." Mason was buried the next day in the post cemetery with full military honors.

"Softening of the brain" is not a diagnosis used nowadays. Apparently, the term originated because some autopsies would show mushiness or bleeding. This was possibly caused by a stroke or hemorrhage, and some medical research indicates it could be caused by advanced syphilis or by encephalitis, inflammation of the brain.

So, as the case of this ex-soldier shows, the U.S. Army did sometimes care for its soldiers who had been discharged for disability. It didn't always just send them home to die after they were no longer fit to be soldiers.

The salary for a soldier (private) was thirteen dollars per month, but one dollar per month was automatically deducted from every soldier's pay to support the Old Soldier's Home in Washington, D.C. Soldiers knew they could go there to live someday, if they needed to. Established in 1851, it has been in continual use since then. It is now known as the Armed Forces Retirement Home.

**FACTOID** Army doctors on the frontier were often the only physician for hundreds of miles. They treated not only military personnel and families but also area civilians.

## Further Reading

Coffman, *Old Army*, 385.
Rickey, *Forty Miles a Day on Beans and Hay*.
U.S. Army, Medical Records, Fort Davis.

## CHAPTER 44

# WHY DID THE U.S. ARMY DELIBERATELY BURN DOWN ITS HOSPITALS?

Until the nineteenth century, hospitals in general had a reputation for being places where disease ran rampant—therefore, most people avoided them. Hospitals tended to be as much charitable or custodial institutions as medical facilities. Mainly, the people admitted were indigent, insane, orphans, disabled, criminals, prostitutes, aged poor or chronically ill, or they had pestilential diseases. It was common knowledge that it was healthier to stay out of hospitals. Home medical care was the preferred treatment. Well-to-do people customarily had the doctor make sick calls to their homes, or they visited the physician's office.

Disease—and what caused disease—was poorly understood. In the early to mid-nineteenth century, the U.S. Army typically burned down a permanent hospital after ten years because it was considered to be thoroughly contaminated with disease. The fail-safe way to control disease: simply burn down the hospital and build a new one!

By the time of America's Civil War, the practice of burning down army hospitals after ten years had stopped. New ways to control disease were emerging—that is, to design hospitals with big windows and doors to allow circulation of lots of fresh air, and to locate hospitals away from people. The army started planning hospital buildings with wards that allowed plenty of space for air to circulate around each bed.

**FACTOID** U.S. Army physician Dr. William Cline Borden, born in 1858, was a graduate of George Washington University School of Medicine in Washington, D.C. He was in his early thirties when he served as the last post surgeon at Fort Davis before the army closed the garrison in 1891. He and his wife, Jennie, had two sons, born in 1887 and 1890.

In the 1880s, the assistant surgeon general reprimanded Dr. Borden to "quit fooling around with the microscope and do things for the [Hospital Medical] Corps"—since spending so much time with the microscope would get him nowhere! Borden, who had a personal interest in microscopic anatomy, or histology, responded that he tended to all his medical duties and still had a lot of spare time, so why not work with the microscope "in place of cards, drinking, hunting, or the club."

As it turned out, the microscope was a crucial tool that fostered progress and aided the new science of bacteriology in unraveling the mysteries of disease causation and transmission. Borden was a close friend of Dr. Walter Reed who did breakthrough research on yellow fever and who died at age fifty-one of appendicitis in 1902. Borden later became a driving force in the establishment in 1909 of Walter Reed Army Medical Center.

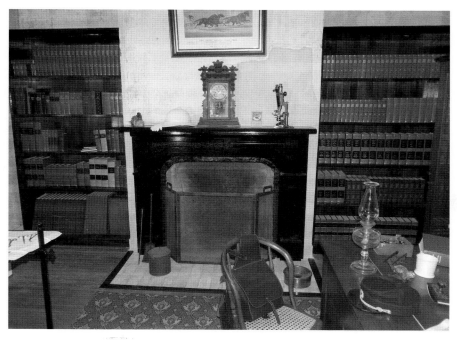

Post surgeon's office at Fort Davis with microscope on mantel. Dr. William Borden served as the last post surgeon at Fort Davis. *Photo by Max Kandler.*

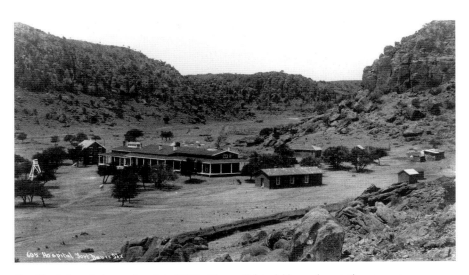

Fort Davis hospital complex, late 1880s. Shows (*left to right*) weather station, two-story hospital steward's quarters, hospital, storeroom, laundry behind. *Lauderdale, Yale University, Beinecke Library.*

When visiting the frontier army post of Fort Davis, you notice it is a trek to get to the post hospital. That far-removed location was deliberate. The hospital's huge windows go almost from floor to ceiling, and the building design allows for air circulation under the floors—typical of army hospitals at the time.

So, a walk of five hundred yards to the Fort Davis Post Hospital makes sense when you put it in the context of nineteenth-century understanding of disease control. The army located this hospital at the mouth of the canyon to take advantage of the breezes to help suppress disease. That was the prevailing state of the art of medicine in America and the world at the time.

Meanwhile, in Europe, scientists and physicians were starting to uncover the mysteries of what caused disease. Not miasmas, bad air or foul vapors rising from the earth, and not poisons in the blood that needed to be released through bloodletting—but microorganisms like bacteria or other pathogens that could not be seen with the naked eye.

Drastic changes were coming to medicine at the end of the nineteenth century. These new concepts would change history. It was the dawn of the age of germ theory.

## *Further Reading*

Ashburn, *History of the Medical Department of the United States Army* [1929], 132, 147–48.

Gillett, *Army Medical Department, 1865–1917* and *Army Medical Department, 1818–1865.*

# GLOSSARY OF OLD MEDICAL TERMS USED IN THE NINETEENTH CENTURY

**Adenitis:** inflammation of a gland; bubo

**Ague:** malaria/remitting fever/chillblains

**Aphonia:** laryngitis

**Apoplexy:** paralysis due to stroke; gross hemorrhage

**Bilious fever:** typhus/typhoid fever

**Biliousness:** jaundice associated with liver disease

**Bladder in throat:** diphtheria

**Bloody flux:** bloody stools

**Brain fever:** meningitis

**Cachexy:** malnutrition

**Canine madness:** rabies

**Catarrh:** a common cold in the head or chest

**Cerebritis:** inflammation of brain or lead poisoning

**Childbed fever:** *see* "puerperal fever"; major cause of maternal mortality when women gave birth in hospitals where attendants did not yet recognize the importance of hygiene and antisepsis

**Chin cough:** whooping cough

**Cholelithiasis:** gall stones

**Cholera:** a vomiting and purging of bile with painful griping and spasm of muscles of the abdomen, calves of the legs, etc.

**Cholera Asiatic:** epidemic disease; severe rapid symptoms ("copious diarrhea, torment of the bowels, vomiting of humor and yellow bile, dangerous fluid loss"); generally fatal

**Cholera infantum:** diarrhea common among small children in summer; attended with vomiting mixed with slime or blood

**Cholera morbus:** nonepidemic cholera; also called European cholera; characterized by severe diarrhea, spasmodic pain, griping of the bowels and sometimes vomiting; could be appendicitis

**Consumption:** any wasting away of the body, but generally applied to pthisis pulmonalis (pulmonary tuberculosis), often fatal

**Coryza:** a "limpy," ropy, mucous defluxion from the nostrils; common cold

**Costiveness:** constipation

**Cramp colic:** appendicitis

**Dropsy:** accumulation of water or fluid; aka congestive heart failure

**Dry bellyache:** lead poisoning

**Emetic:** agent used to induce vomiting

**Epistaxis:** bleeding from the nose

**Erysipelas:** redness or inflammation of skin, with fever and vesications (blisters); contagious; called St. Anthony's Fire

**Falling sickness:** epilepsy

**Fistula in ano:** a fistula (tunnel/cavity) in the cellular substance about the anus or rectum

**Flux:** diarrhea/dysentery

**French pox/great pox:** syphilis

**Furuncle:** boil or inflammatory tumor; a blain

**Gathering:** a collection of pus

**Germ theory:** the theory that many diseases are caused by tiny microorganisms known as pathogens or "germs"; in the late 1800s, this theory gradually revolutionized the practice of medicine

**Glandular fever:** mononucleosis

**Gleet:** thin matter issuing out of ulcers, generally a result of gonorrheal disease

**Gravel:** kidney stone(s)

**Green fever or green sickness:** anemia

**Grippe/grip/la grippe:** influenza or influenza symptoms

**Herpes circintus:** ringworm

**Icterus:** jaundice; yellowness of skin and eyes

**Lead poisoning:** common because lead salts were used in medicines before the dangers were understood, and workers were exposed to lead; causes nerve and brain damage, anemia, blue line on gums, mental disorders

**Lockjaw:** tetanus

**Long sickness:** tuberculosis

**Lumbago:** rheumatic affection of the muscles about the loins; *see* rheumatism

**Lumbricoides:** long, round worm found in the intestines

**Lung fever:** pneumonia

**Lung sickness:** tuberculosis

**Malingerer:** one who simulates or feigns disease to avoid labor or punishment

**Materia medica:** collectively, all the drugs or curative substances used in medicine

**Miasmas:** poisonous, foul odors arising from the earth believed to infect the air and cause disease; the "miasma theory" was commonly accepted until the late 1800s when "germ theory" began to be accepted

**Milk leg:** thrombophlebitis; postpartum blood clots that sometimes caused death

**Nostalgia:** homesickness; melancholia; aka soldier's heart; symptoms of sleeplessness and anxiety; term sometimes used by medical personnel for what was identified many years later (circa 1980) as post-traumatic stress disorder

**Parotitis:** mumps; inflammation of parotid gland

**Phlegmon:** a bright red inflammation

**Phthisis:** tuberculosis of the lungs; characterized by emaciation, debility, cough, hectic fever and purulent expectoration

**Podagra:** gout

**Puerperal exhaustion:** death due to childbirth

**Puerperal fever/childbed fever:** infection of the mother following birth of a child

**Pyrexia:** fever

**Quinsy:** tonsillitis; severe sore throat

**Rheumatism (Screws):** any disorder associated with pain in joints

**Rose cold:** hay fever or nasal symptoms of an allergy

**Rubeola:** measles

**Sciatica:** rheumatism in the hips

**Softening of the brain:** could be cerebral hemorrhage, stroke, dementia, perhaps multiple sclerosis or Parkinson's

**Vaccinia/vaccina:** cowpox, a disease originating in the cow; the human body, if inoculated with it, will be preserved from the contagion of smallpox; also called variola vaccina

**Varicella:** chicken pox

**Variola:** smallpox

**Virus:** something that causes a disease; cannot survive outside the body (term first used in 1728, but not until the 1880s were viruses identified as microorganisms; during the Civil War, the most significant viruses were measles and smallpox)

**Whitlow:** abscess near the nail of the fingers

**Winter Fever:** pneumonia

**Womb Fever:** infection of the uterus

## *Further Reading*

Billings, *National Medical Dictionary*, 1890.

Flint, *Principles and Practice of Medicine*, 1866.

Foster, *Illustrated Encyclopaedic Medical Dictionary*, 1888.

Thomas, *Comprehensive Medical Dictionary*, 1872.

# EXCERPTS FROM FORT DAVIS MILITARY DEATH RECORDS

| Name | Rank | Company or Regiment | Cause of Death | Age | Date |
|------|------|---------------------|----------------|-----|------|
| Reuben Coleman | SGT | 9th U.S. Cavalry | Dysentery | – | 8-14-1867 |
| Shadrach Martin | PVT | 9th U.S. Cavalry | Cerebro meningitis | – | 3-19-1868 |
| Frank Roach | PVT | 9th U.S. Cavalry | Pericardites [sic] | – | 4-28-1868 |
| William Asberry | PVT | 9th U.S. Cavalry | Scurvy | 20 | 6-1-1868 |
| Oliver Johnson | PVT | 9th U.S. Cavalry | Scurvy | 22 | 7-1-1868 |
| Henry Williams | PVT | 41st U.S. Infantry | Dysentery | 27 | 8-6-1868 |
| Henry Butler | PVT | 41st U.S. Infantry | Heart disease | 35 | 7-7-1869 |
| Frank Glenn | PVT | 24th U.S. Infantry | Inflammation of lungs | 26 | 5-15-1871 |
| George W. Harris | PVT | 9th U.S. Cavalry | Dysentery | 25 | 8-30-1872 |
| George A. Brown | PVT | Band, 25th U.S. Infantry | Dysentery | 23 | 9-18-1872 |
| Eli Smallgood | PVT | 25th U.S. Infantry | Consumption | 28 | 11-2-1872 |

| Name | Rank | Company or Regiment | Cause of Death | Age | Date |
|---|---|---|---|---|---|
| James Hill Patterson | CAPT | 25th U.S. Infantry | Acute articular rheumatism | 30 | 8-19-1873 |
| John Holcher | ORD SGT | 9th U.S. Cavalry / 25th U.S. Infantry | Rheumatism | 35 | 9-17-1873 |
| George Patrick | PVT | 9th U.S. Cavalry | Consumption | 21 | 7-5-1874 |
| Patrick Kelliher | LIEUT | 25th U.S. Infantry | Consumption | 28 | 2-12-1876 |
| George Wilson | PVT | 25th U.S. Infantry | Accidental discharge while cleaning his weapon | 22 | 7-19-1876 |
| Abram Jackson | CPL | 25th U.S. Infantry | Murdered 3 miles from Fort Davis | 36 | 11-11-1876 |
| James Lusk | PVT | 25th U.S. Infantry | Inflammation of lungs | 24 | 1-30-1877 |
| Toby Powell | PVT | 25th U.S. Infantry | Dropsy | 28 | 5-10-1877 |
| John Lisly/Lisby | PVT | 10th U.S. Cavalry | Typhoid fever | 27 | 6-29-1877 |
| John M. Morgan | PVT | 10th U.S. Cavalry | Shot by sentry when trying to rob post bakery | 22 | 11-27-1877 |
| Richard Robinson | CPL | 25th U.S. Infantry | Killed by his sergeant | 31 | 6-13-1878 |
| Solomon Mapp | PVT | 25th U.S. Infantry | Drowned crossing flooded Limpia Creek in a wagon | 29 | 10-10-1879 |
| William Myers | PVT | 10th U.S. Cavalry | Smallpox— died in isolated hospital tent | 24 | 10-26-879 |

| Name | Rank | Company or Regiment | Cause of Death | Age | Date |
|------|------|---------------------|----------------|-----|------|
| Benjamin Small/ Smalley | PVT | 10th U.S. Cavalry | Consumption —died after 2 months in hospital; autopsy done; lungs sent to Army Medical Museum in D.C. | 24 | 3-23-1880 |
| Martin Davis | PVT | 10th U.S. Cavalry | KIA with Apaches | 22 | 7-30-1880 |
| Henry Miller | PVT | 16th U.S. Infantry | Accidentally shot while serving as paymaster escort | | 9-4-1880 |
| Albert Christopher | PVT | 10th U.S. Cavalry | Obstruction of bowel | 28 | 4- 8-1881 |
| Rafael Ortiz | PVT | 1st U.S. Infantry | Pneumonia | 21/ 22 | 4-9-1881 |
| John S. Mitchell | PVT | 10th U.S. Cavalry | Internal injuries from horse kick in abdomen | 22 | 7-9-1881 |
| Everett Thomas | PVT | 10th U.S. Cavalry | Consumption | 28 | 7-18-1881 |
| James F. Holmes | PVT | 1st U.S. Infantry | Gunshot wound, accidental | 22 | 9-27-1881 |
| John Gaddess | PVT | 10th U.S. Cavalry | Pneumonia | 40 | 11-25-1882 |
| Dorsey Johnson | PVT | 10th U.S. Cavalry | Pneumonia | 24 | 3-5-1883 |
| Wesley Lane | PVT | 10th U.S. Cavalry | Chronic inflammation of lungs | 36 | 10-2-1883 |

| Name | Rank | Company or Regiment | Cause of Death | Age | Date |
|------|------|---------------------|----------------|-----|------|
| James Gardner | PVT | 10th U.S. Cavalry | Remittent fever | 37 | 11-18-1884 |
| Benjamin Banks | PVT | 10th U.S. Cavalry | Acute dysentery | 23 | 11-25-1884 |
| Henry C. Beresford | PVT | 16th U.S. Infantry | Inflammation of brain (cerebritis) | 34 | 12-5-1884 |
| John H. Mason | Ex-CPL | 10th U.S. Cavalry | Softening of the brain | 38 | 6-29-1886 |
| John Gunning | PVT | 16th U.S. Infantry | Peritonitis | 27 | 10-12-1886 |
| Charles Schurtz | PVT | 3rd U.S. Cavalry | Typhoid fever | 22 | 10-15-1886 |
| Patrick J. McGill | PVT | 3rd U.S. Cavalry | Drowned in Rio Grande on patrol | 21 | 7-8-1887 |
| Michael Arbogast | PVT | 3rd U.S. Cavalry | Liver abscess | 25 | 7-16-1887 |
| James Powers | PVT | 5th U.S. Infantry | Meningitis | 50 | 8-5-1890 |
| Patrick Delmar | PVT | 5th U.S. Infantry | Suicide | 31 | 4-9-1891 |

# BIBLIOGRAPHY

AMEDD (U.S. Army Medical Department) Museum (San Antonio, TX). https://armymedicalmuseum.org/

Ancestry.com.

Arlington National Cemetery (Arlington, VA). www.arlingtoncemetery.mil

Army Medical Museum (former name for what is now called the National Museum of Health and Medicine, Silver Spring, MD). https://medicalmuseum.health.mil/

Ashurn, P[ercy] M. *History of the Medical Department of the United States Army.* Boston: Houghton Mifflin, 1929.

Baldwin, Alice Blackwood. *Memoirs of the Late Major Frank D. Baldwin.* Los Angeles: Wetzel Publishing, 1929.

Barthelmess, Casey. *Photographer on an Army Mule.* Norman: University of Oklahoma Press, 1965.

Bartholow, Roberts. *Practical Treatise on Materia Medica and Therapeutics.* New York: Appleton, 1876.

Biddle, Ellen McGowan. *Reminiscences of a Soldier's Wife.* Philadelphia: Lippincott, 1907.

Bigelow, John Jr. *Garrison Tangles in the Friendless Tenth: Journal of First Lieutenant John Bigelow, Jr., Fort Davis, Texas,* ed. Douglas C. McChristian. Bryan, TX: J.M. Carroll, 1985.

Bill, J[oseph] H[owland]. "Forceps for the Extraction of Arrow-Heads." *Medical Record: A Weekly Journal of Medicine & Surgery* 11 (April 8, 1876), ed. George F. Shrady. New York: William Wood, 1876.

Billings, John Shaw. *The National Medical Dictionary*, 2 vols. Philadelphia: Lea Bros., 1890.

Bishop, David (great-grandson of Mattie Howell Adams Collins Bishop). Author interview, 2019. Fairfax City, VA.

Blanton, DeAnne, and Lauren M. Cook. *They Fought Like Demons: Women Soldiers in the American Civil War.* Baton Rouge: Louisiana State University Press, 2002.

Bluthardt, Robert F. "Baseball on the Military Frontier." *Fort Concho Report* 19 (Spring 1987). Fort Concho National Historic Landmark, San Angelo, TX.

Bynum, W.F. *Science and the Practice of Medicine.* Cambridge: Cambridge University Press, 1994.

Calcaterra, Nicholas. "4-F: Unfit for Service Because of Your Teeth?" Directions in Dentistry website, March 19, 2013.

Cantwell, Emma Dutchover (descendant of George and Concepcion Bentley). Fort Davis, TX. Author interview, 2019.

Carriker, Robert C. and Eleanor R., eds. *An Army Wife on the Frontier: The Memoirs of Alice Blackwood Baldwin, 1867–1877.* Salt Lake City: Tanner Trust Fund, University of Utah Library, 1975.

Carter, K. Codell, and Barbara R. Carter. *Childbed Fever: A Scientific Biography of Ignaz Semmelweis.* New Jersey and London: Transaction Publishers, 2005.

Centers for Disease Control and Prevention. "Table 15. Life Expectancy at Birth, at Age 65, and at Age 75, by Sex, Race, and Hispanic Origin: United States, Selected Years 1900–2014." www.cdc.gov/nchs/

Clary, David A. "The Role of the Army Surgeon in the West: Daniel Weisel at Fort Davis, Texas, 1868–1872," *Western Historical Quarterly* (January 1972).

Coe, Alexis. "Mary Walker's Quest to Be Appointed as a Union Doctor in the Civil War." *Atlantic,* February 7, 2013.

Coffman, Edward M. *The Old Army.* New York: Oxford University Press, 1986.

Craig, Stephen C. *In the Interest of Truth: The Life and Science of Surgeon General George Miller Sternberg.* Fort Sam Houston, TX: Office of Surgeon General, Borden Institute, U.S. Army Medical Department and School, 2013.

Dart, Richard (grandson of Rachel and hospital steward Richard Dart). Author interview, 2007. Carlsbad, NM; subsequent communication with Michael Kennedy (great-grandson of Dart) in Colorado.

Deglman, Frank, and Donna G. Smith. "Roll Call of the Dead: An Accounting of Army Deaths at Fort Davis, Texas 1854–1891," *Journal of Big Bend Studies* 26 (2014). Alpine, TX: Sul Ross State University.

Dixon, Ann. "Letters from Texas: An Army Wife on the Texas Frontier 1856–1860," *Journal of Big Bend Studies* 26 (2014). Sul Ross State University, Alpine, TX.

Eales, Anne Bruner. *Living Within the Sound of Bugles: Army Wives on the American Frontier.* Boulder, CO: Johnson Books, 1996.

EyeWitness to History.com. "Baseball Glove Comes to Baseball, 1875." 2004. www.eyewitnesstohistory.com/baseball.htm

FamilySearch. www.familysearch.org

Find a Grave. www.findagrave.com

Fisher, Barbara E., ed. "Forrestine Cooper Hooker's Notes and Memoirs on Army Life in the West, 1871–1876." Master's thesis, University of Arizona, 1963.

FitzGerald, Emily McCorkle. *An Army Doctor's Wife on the Frontier: The Letters of Emily McCorkle FitzGerald from Alaska and the Far West, 1874–1878,* ed. Abe Laufe. Pittsburgh: University of Pittsburgh Press, 1962.

Flint, Austin. *Treatise on the Principles and Practice of Medicine.* Philadelphia: Henry C. Lea, 1866.

Fort Davis National Historic Site archival library.

Foster, Frank P. *An Illustrated Encyclopaedic Medical Dictionary*, 4 vols. New York: Appleton, 1888.

Fougera, Katherine Gibson. *With Custer's Cavalry.* Lincoln: University of Nebraska Press, 1986. First published 1942.

Gillett, Mary C. *The Army Medical Department, 1818–1865.* Washington, D.C.: U.S. Army Center of Military History, 1987.

———. *The Army Medical Department, 1865–1917.* Washington, D.C.: U.S. Army Center of Military History, 1995.

Glisan, Rodney. *Journal of Army Life.* San Francisco: A.L. Bancroft, 1874.

Graf, Mercedes. *A Woman of Honor: Dr. Mary E. Walker and the Civil War.* Gettysburg, PA: Thomas Publications, 2001.

Green, Bill. *The Dancing Was Lively—Fort Concho, Texas: A Social History 1867 to 1882.* San Angelo, TX: Fort Concho Sketches Publishing Company, 1974.

Greene, Jerome A. *Historic Resource Study: Fort Davis National Historic Site.* Denver, CO: National Park Service, 1986.

Gross, S[amuel] D[avid]. *A Manual of Military Surgery; or, Hints on the Emergencies of Field, Camp, and Hospital Practice.* San Francisco: Norman Publishing, 1988. First published 1861 by J.B. Lippincott (Philadelphia).

Hardy, Anne. *The Epidemic Streets: Infectious Disease and the Rise of Preventive Medicine, 1856–1900.* Oxford: Clarendon, 1993.

Harman, S.W. *Hell on the Border*, comp. C.P. Sterns. Fort Smith, AR: Phoenix Publishing, 1898.

Harvey, O.F. (army surgeon). *Fort Buford Medical Report*. October 6, 1878.

Hastings, Paul. *Medicine: An International History*. New York: Praeger, 1974.

Heitman, Francis Bernard. *Historical Register and Dictionary of the United States Army*. Washington, D.C.: GPO, 1903.

Hooker, Forrestine C[ooper]. *Child of the Fighting Tenth: On the Frontier with the Buffalo Soldiers*, ed. Steve Wilson. New York: Oxford University Press, 2003.

Hume, Edgar Erskine. *Ornithologists of the United States Army Medical Corps: 36 Biographies*. Baltimore, MD: Johns Hopkins Press, 1942.

Ifera, Raymond Philip. "Crime and Punishment, 1867–1891." Master's thesis, Sul Ross State University, 1974.

Jacobson, Lucy Miller, and Mildred Bloys Nored. *Jeff Davis County, Texas*. Fort Davis, TX: Fort Davis Historical Society, 1993.

Lauderdale, John Vance. Papers and "Letterbooks, 1885–1892, Vols. 8–9." Yale University Collection of Americana, Beinecke Rare Book and Manuscript Library, New Haven, CT.

Lawrence, Jennifer J. *Soap Suds Row: Bold Lives of Army Laundresses, 1820–1878*. Glendo, WY: High Plains Press, 2016.

Leckie, Shirley A., ed. *The Colonel's Lady on the Western Frontier: The Correspondence of Alice Kirk Grierson*. Lincoln: University of Nebraska Press, 1989.

Leiker, James N. "George Goldsby," in *Soldiers in the Southwest Borderlands 1848–1886*, ed. Janne Lahti. Norman: University of Oklahoma Press, 2017.

Lindley, John Patterson (great-grandson of Captain James Hill Patterson; Bradley, CA). Communication with author, 2002 to present.

Lineberry, Cate. "I Wear My Own Clothes," editorial, *New York Times*, December 2, 2013.

Malburne, Meredith. "Susie King Taylor, b. 1848." Documenting the American South. University Library, The University of North Carolina at Chapel Hill. https://docsouth.unc.edu

Major General Frank D. Baldwin Collection. Mossey Library Special Collections, Hillsdale College, Hillsdale, Michigan.

Medical History of Fort Buford, Dakota Territory.

Metheny, Hannah. "'For a Woman': The Fight for Civil War Army Nurses." Undergraduate honors thesis, College of William and Mary, 2013. Paper 573.

Miller, Darlis A. "Foragers, Army Women, and Prostitutes," in *New Mexico Women: Intercultural Perspectives*, ed. Joan M. Jensen and Darlis A. Miller. Albuquerque: University of New Mexico Press, 1986.

Mills, Anson. *My Story*, ed. C.H. Claudy. 2nd ed. Washington, D.C.: Press of Byron S. Adams, 1921.

Mohr, James C. *Abortion in America: Origins and Evolution of National Policy, 1800–1900*. New York: Oxford University, 1978.

Mulford, [Private] Ami Frank. *Fighting Indians! In The Seventh United States Cavalry, Custer's Favorite Regiment*. Fairfield, WA: Ye Galleon Press, 1972.

Museum of Health Care at Kingston. "Diphtheria" (for Princess Alice information). http://www.museumofhealthcare.ca

Myres, Sandra L., ed. "A Woman's View of the Texas Frontier, 1874: Diary of Emily K. Andrews." Texas State Historical Association, *Southwestern Historical Quarterly* 86, July 1982–April 1983. Original at Dolph Briscoe Center, UT, Austin.

———. *Ho for California! Women's Overland Diaries from Huntington Library*. San Marino, CA: Huntington Library, 1980.

National Museum of Civil War Medicine (Frederick, MD). www.civilwarmed.org.

National Park Service. "Dr. Mary Edwards Walker." https://www.nps.gov/people/mary-walker.htm

———. "Letter Regarding Widow Pension Request, Jan. 1884." https://www.nps.gov/fols/learn/historyculture/telegram-reporting-nolan-death.htm

*New York Times*. Obituary of Dr. Mary Edwards Walker. February 23, 1919.

Nored, Mildred, and Jane Wiant. *Early Homes and Buildings of Fort Davis, Texas 1855–1929*. Fort Davis, TX: Bloys Books, 1997.

Oliva, Leo E. *Fort Union and the Frontier Army in the Southwest*. Southwest Cultural Resource Center Professional Papers No. 41. Santa Fe, NM: National Park Service, 1993.

Oswego State University of New York. Biography of Dr. Mary Edwards Walker. Special Collections. libraryguides.oswego.edu

Overland Trail Museum (511 Fort Street, Fort Davis, TX). Operated by the Fort Davis Historical Society.

Parker, W. Thornton, ed. *Records of the Association of Acting Assistant Surgeons of the United States Army*. Salem, MA: Salem Press, 1891.

Pernick, Martin S. *A Calculus of Suffering: Pain, Professionalism, and Anesthesia in Nineteenth-Century America*. New York: Columbia University Press, 1985.

Prucha, Francis Paul. *A Guide to the Military Posts of the United States, 1789–1895*. Madison, WI: State Historical Society, 1964.

Quebbeman, Frances E. *Medicine in Territorial Arizona*. Phoenix: Arizona Historical Foundation, 1966.

Reeder, Red [Russell Potter]. *Born at Reveille.* New York: Duell, Sloan & Pearce: 1966.

Reimer, Terry (director of research at the National Museum of Civil War Medicine). "Anesthesia in Civil War." National Museum of Civil War Medicine online.

————. Communication with author about blue mass pills.

Rickey, Don Jr. *Forty Miles a Day on Beans and Hay.* Norman: University of Oklahoma Press, 1963.

RootsWeb. https://home.rootsweb.com/

Rothstein, William G. *American Physicians in the 19th Century: From Sects to Science.* Baltimore, MD: Johns Hopkins Press, 1972.

San Antonio National Cemetery. https://www.cem.va.gov/cems/nchp/SanAntonio.asp

Sauerwein, Daniel (reference specialist at State Historical Society of North Dakota, Bismarck). Communication with author, 2018.

Sayre, Harold. *Warriors of Color.* Fort Davis, TX: self-published, 1995.

Sitka History Museum. "Letters from Emily [McCorkle FitzGerald]." sitkahistory.com.

Smith, Donna Gerstle. "Army Physicians, Nineteenth Century Medicine, the U.S. Army Medical Department, and 1880s Medical Care of the Sick and Injured at Fort Davis, Texas." Master's thesis; Sul Ross State University, Alpine, TX; 1997.

————. "Till Death or Discharge Do Us Part: The State of Medicine at the Nineteenth Century U.S. Army Post of Fort Davis, Texas." *Journal of Big Bend Studies* 25 (2013). Sul Ross State University, Alpine, TX.

Smith, Ralph Adam. *Borderlander: The Life of James Kirker, 1793–1852.* Norman: University of Oklahoma Press, 1999.

Smith, Thomas T., Jerry D. Thompson, Robert Wooster and Ben E. Pingenot. *The Reminiscences of Major General Zenas R. Bliss, 1854–1876.* Austin: Texas State Historical Association, 2007.

Sobel, Dava. *Longitude: The Story of a Lone Genius Who Solved the Greatest Scientific Problem of His Time.* New York: Walker Publishing, 1995.

Stacey, May Humphreys, Edward Fitzgerald Beale and Lewis Burt Lesley. *Uncle Sam's Camels: The Journal of May Humphreys Stacey Supplemented by the Report of Edward Fitzgerald Beale (1857–1858).* Cambridge: Harvard University Press, 1929.

Stallard, Patricia Y. *Glittering Misery: Dependents of the Indian Fighting Army.* Fort Collins, CO: Old Army Press, 1978.

Steinbach, Robert H. *A Long March: The Lives of Frank and Alice Baldwin.* Austin: University of Texas Press, 1989.

Stewart, Miller J. "Army Laundresses: Ladies of Soap Suds Row." *Nebraska History* 61 (Winter 1980).

Summerhayes, Martha. *Vanished Arizona.* Chicago: Lakeside Press, R.R. Donnelley & Sons, 1939.

Tavernier, Robert. "Major John Conline, 1846–1916." Michigan Commandery Military Order of the Loyal Legion of the United States; also Sons of Union Veterans of Civil War.

Taylor, Susie King. *Reminiscences of My Life in Camp with the 33d United States Colored Troops, Late 1ˢᵗ S.C. Volunteers.* Boston, MA: self-published, 1902.

Texas State Library and Archives Commission. "Texas State Penitentiary Convict Records: Moses Marshall." Austin, TX.

Thomas, Joseph. *Comprehensive Medical Dictionary.* Philadelphia: Lippincott, 1872.

Thompson, Cecilia. *History of Marfa and Presidio County, Texas, 1535–1946.* Austin, TX: Nortex Press, 1985.

Thrapp, Dan L. *Encyclopedia of Frontier Biography*, vol. 2. Spokane, WA: Arthur H. Clark, 1990.

Tiemann, George, & Co. (corporate author). *American Armamentarium Chirurgicum.* New York: C.H. Ludwig, 1889. Republished by Norman Pub, San Francisco and the Printers' Devil, Boston, 1989.

U.S. Army. Hospital Registers. All U.S. Army records cited are preserved at the National Archives.

———. Medical History of Posts.

———. Medical Records.

———. Personal Papers of Medical Officers and Physicians (MOP).

———. Records of Adjutant General's Office—Registers of the Sick and Wounded.

———. Records of Appointment, Commission, and Personal (ACP) Branch.

———. Records of Chief of Engineers.

———. Records of Hospital Stewards.

———. Records of Inspector General.

———. Records of Quartermaster General.

———. Records of Record and Pension Office.

———. Records of Surgeon General.

———. Records of U.S. Army Continental Command.

———. Regimental Returns.

———. Registers of Patients.

———. Returns of Matrons.

U.S. Census Bureau. 1860 Census.

———. 1870 Census.

———. 1880 Census.

U.S. Department of Veterans Affairs, National Cemetery Administration. https://gravelocator.cem.va.gov/ngl/index.jsp

U.S. War Department. *Regulations of the Army of the United States and General Orders in Force on the 17th of February, 1881.* Washington, D.C.: Government Printing Office, 1881.

———. *Standard Supply Table of the Medical Department of the United States Army, 1871.* Bethesda, MD: National Library of Medicine.

———. *Standard Supply Table of the Medical Department of the United States Army, 1883.* Bethesda, MD: National Library of Medicine.

Walker, Mary Edwards. Medal of Honor, 1974–77. Bobbie Greene Kilberg Files, Gerald R. Ford Presidential Library. Online at www.fordlibrarymuseum.gov/library

Weigley, Russell F. *History of the United States Army.* New York: Macmillan, 1967.

Williams, Mary L. "Care of the Dead: A Neglected Duty; The Military Cemeteries at Fort Davis, Texas," September 15, 1983. Unpublished research paper. Available at the Fort Davis National Historic Site library archives.

Woodward, Joseph Janvier, MD. *The Hospital Steward's Manual.* Philadelphia: J.B. Lippincott, 1862.

Wooster, Robert. *Frontier Crossroads: Fort Davis and the West.* College Station: Texas A&M University Press, 2006.

———. *History of Fort Davis, Texas.* Southwest Cultural Resources Center Professional Papers No. 34. Santa Fe, NM: National Park Service, 1990.

Wright, Fred P. Biographical paper on Dr. Mary Walker given May 19, 1953, to Oswego County Historical Society. Ford Presidential Library Archives, Bobbie Greene Kilberg Files, Ann Arbor, Michigan. https://www.fordlibrarymuseum.gov

# INDEX

Mills, Major Anson; wife Hannah Cassel 67, 121

Mitchell, James Livingston (Twenty-Ninth Iowa Volunteer Infantry); second wife Elizabeth Vandegrift Patterson; son Frank 33

morphine/morphia 89, 110, 124, 126

Mulford, Private Ami Frank (Seventh U.S. Cavalry) 100–101, 148–149

Mullins, George G. (post chaplain) 151

Murphy, Sergeant James (Third U.S. Cavalry); son James 120

Myer, Albert James, MD 56

**N**

Native Americans/Native people(s) 18, 31, 36, 43, 66, 87, 97, 131, 132, 143

Navajo 141

Nez Perce 76, 148

Nocona, Peta (Comanche chief); wife Cynthia Ann Parker; son Quanah Parker 29

Nolan, Captain Nicholas; wives Annie M. Sullivan and Anne Eleanor Dwyer 140, 141

**O**

Old Soldiers' Home (Washington, D.C.; now called Armed Forces Retirement Home) 157–159

opium 46, 71, 89, 101, 120, 121, 126

Otis, Colonel Elmer 127, 129

**P**

Parker, Quanah 29, 31

Pasteur, Louis (born in France, 1822) 25, 80, 83, 87

patent medicine 36, 120

Patterson, Captain James Hill (Twenty-Fifth U.S. Infantry); wife Elizabeth Ellen Vandegrift (later Mitchell); son John Love 32–34, 112, 170

pay (salary) of enlisted men, officers, laundresses 55, 56, 64, 67, 99, 104, 159

pensions 28, 64, 77, 138
  widow's pensions 26, 33, 76, 141

Peters, DeWitt Clinton, MD; wife Emily 56

peyote 18, 29–31

photography 41–44
  postmortem 115

Picotte, Susan La Flesche, MD 139

Pilcher, James Elijah, MD 125

Pioneer Cemetery (town of Fort Davis) 25

pneumonia 76, 85, 110, 125, 167, 168, 171

post-traumatic stress disorder 149

Powers, Michael (Eighth U.S. Infantry) 19

Pratt, Private John (Eighth U.S. Infantry) 19

prisoner of war 55, 86, 95, 97, 138

Pruett, Will 102

# ABOUT THE AUTHOR

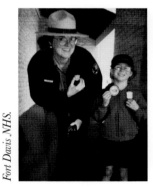

Donna Gerstle Smith worked for the National Park Service for almost three decades as park ranger and park historian. Her fascination with history began while researching for her master's degree thesis on nineteenth-century medicine at frontier military posts, especially Fort Davis. Inspired by reading old letters, journals, army medical records and other primary source materials, she found them to be priceless windows for looking into the past. As she says, "It was like time stopped! I walked through a door and met real people, long dead now, whose lives were full of emotion, tragedy, adventure and challenges—just like ours."

THE AUTHOR IS A preeminent historian, inviting readers to join her on a journey. These are true-to-life narratives of sickness, love and heartache, told with candor and compassion. People at army forts in the West who lived, suffered and sometimes died—their stories are too good to be forgotten, treasures filled with historical richness. Some accounts are unforgettable, some are humorous, some are almost incredible—but all are true. Reading them will take you on a remarkable trip. Some will make your jaw drop; some will bring you to tears. This is history that's vibrant and intriguing. It's untold stories. It's authentic history sure to touch readers' hearts.

*Visit us at*
www.historypress.com
···················································